Animal Teachings

from
Hayley's Angels Methods

Joanne Lefebvre, DVM

WingSpan Press

Printed in the United States of America
Published by WingSpan Press, Livermore, CA
www.wingspanpress.com
The WingSpan name, logo and colophon
are the trademarks of WingSpan Publishing.

First Edition 2011

ISBN 978-1-59594-446-7

Library of Congress Control Number: 2011937508

This book is printed on 20% post-consumer, acid-free paper
Publisher's Cataloging-in-Publication Data
Lefebvre, Joanne.
Animal Teachings from Hayley's Angels Methods/Joanne Lefebvre.
p. cm.
1. Human-animal communication. 3. Human-animal relationships.
2. Pets—Death—Psychological aspects. I. Title.
SF411.47 .L39 2011
.9`37155—dc22
2011937508

This book is printed on 20% post-consumer, acid-free paper

During the turn of the New Year 2011, I became surrounded by a strong whale energy that lasted about two weeks. My soul experienced several moments of swimming with those powerful creatures which hold so much wisdom. Each meditative session would bring me strength and refuge in their reassurance and guidance to reconnect with the Source, as I could feel my body energy shifting, representing the end of a chapter in my life and the beginning of a new one. Their divine guidance brought me peace and comfort during time of spiritual growth, which is exciting but also scary.

I was guided during that time to create two water color paintings. The cover of this book is the first one and represents living in harmony with our world, being in communion with our Universe at all times, with Mother Earth, Father Sky and all of nature's creations and creatures. The second painting is the back of this book. It represents how swimming with the whales helps you stabilize during spiritual growth and shifting of your body's energies. Here is a message from the Whales to everyone on the planet:

Feel the power of my wisdom, Feel my strength
Feel my love & support as your energies are shifting
And vibrating at a higher level of
Divine consciousness
Thank you for contributing to healing our world
x x x x x x x x x x x x x x x x x

Thank you Hayley, sweet girl, for your Heavenly guidance.

Thank you to my faithful furry friends Mocha, Yogi, Sunny and Munchie who have been by my side during the writing of this book.

Thank you to my inner child for these inspiring paintings, thank you to Rebecca and her skilled graphic assistant, Betsy, from Centric Photo, for digitizing them for the book.

Table of Contents

Introduction &
Acknowledgments

Born in Quebec, Canada, I graduated from the University of Montreal Veterinary School in 2001. My training included completing several externships in highly reputable American veterinary schools such as Tufts Veterinary School in Massachusetts, Colorado State University, The Ohio State University, and The College of Veterinary Medicine at Cornell University in New York. After graduation, I was one of the very few selected for a one year-long internship specializing in small animal medicine, surgery, emergency and critical care at Michigan Veterinary Specialists. That year, I published a scientific and clinical study in the British Journal of Small Animal Practice about the use of computed tomography in diagnosing nasal diseases in dogs.

Since then, my life has led me to work at and help several non-profit animal rescue groups and shelters. I have visited over fifty small animal veterinary hospitals across the United States and I have worked at more than thirty hospitals, either full-time or as a relief veterinarian. I have helped dogs, cats, rats, hamsters, rabbits, ferrets, pigs, horses, goats, chickens, ducks, birds, sea otters, bears, raptors, raccoons, insects and the list continues to grow. I am currently licensed to practice as a veterinarian in Quebec, Canada, as well as in California and Arizona, USA, calling Arizona my home for the last six years.

Interestingly enough, a couple of years ago, I was blessed with the opportunity to shadow a medical doctor for humans, as well as talk with medical students during a night-long shift in the emergency room of a large, well-known hospital in the heart of Montreal, Canada. This experience made me realize that, unfortunately, the training that all medical students get in school (in veterinary or human medicine) is sadly limited to help the physical body. No one teaches us how to care for the mind or the soul. Additionally, the medical staff is often overwhelmed by the number of patients, and patients become numbers. Procedures are done "routinely" and we forget that patients only go through the procedure once for the most part and it is therefore not routine to them. Each patient (human or animal) gets scared and anxious, therefore, needs support and reassurance from the medical team. After reading *The Scalpel and the Soul*, a book written by the neurosurgeon Dr. Allan Hamilton, I feel compelled to act in response to the sad state of affairs in modern medical establishments and to the urgency of sharing ideas to improve the care of people and animals worldwide.

I met my husband just a few months after finishing my schooling and I credit him for shaping me into the better person and veterinarian that I am today. With his sensibility towards animals and his heartfelt passion for what he believes in, he has taught me several life-improving secrets. The most important lesson above all is that school fills your brain with a lot of great knowledge, whereas The School of Life shapes your heart emotionally in how to apply this knowledge in the real world to be able to serve humanity to the best of your ability and highest potential. In order to be the best human being and doctor combined, with everlasting care and compassion, you need the perfect balance between the two.

My mother and father have always been present in my life and their support has always been as solid as a rock. My mother is a naturopath and energy healer who has owned a successful health food and spiritual growth shop for over twenty-five years. I have applied a lot of her ideas to the veterinary world. To both my parents, thank you for teaching me that the sky is the limit, for always being supportive of who I am, and supportive of the work that I am here on Earth to accomplish.

In 2007, the transition of our beloved dog Hayley was the beginning of a never expected spiritual journey that is still continuing today, bringing more joy and fulfillment in life than ever. *Hayley's Angels Veterinary Services* has helped over one thousand sick pets have a peaceful transition into the Afterlife, in the comfort of home, surrounded by their family members. *Hayley's Angels Methods* are teaching people worldwide how to better care for animals on their paths, but also how to better care for themselves. Once again, Hayley, thank you sweet girl!!

Just a few months before writing this book, the Universe brought into my life a wave of mediums followed by a wave of authors. Each wave came with feelings that overwhelmed me at first, but were quickly followed by peace and understanding. Strangely, I felt like I was one of them. The next chapter of my life mission was about to begin, with the writing of this book. Why do we (animals and people) get sick? Is there a relationship between emotions, our mind set and our physical body? Does everything happen for a reason? How can we learn from an illness or a difficulty in our life? Do you listen to the signs of guidance in your life to make better decisions? What are Animal Communication and Intuitive Medicine, and how much can they help you and your pet? How can we better care for our physical and emotional bodies, and the ones of our pets? Can we all decide to have a peaceful transition into the next world? What is the Afterlife? Do we all, animals and humans, go to the same place?

I finally want to thank all the animals on my path as well as their human families. Animals ARE the best teachers. As a doctor of animals or humans, one may be resistant at first to learn from his/her patients. However, I am here to suggest to everyone to open up to all the divine teachings that both people and animals are offering you; embrace the rich secrets for happiness and health. Welcoming these teachings will help you experience a deeper sense of fulfillment in realizing your life's purpose. I am excited to share this book with you, drawn from the teachings of the Universe, the Spirit World, Mother Nature and its animals, all who have provided me with selfless guidance. I know they are waiting to teach you as well. Together, it is possible to awaken to a new reality, a new life, a new world and a better place for all humans and animals, based on unconditional love, respect, support, sharing and giving. May this book enlighten you and guide you into leading a blissful life here on Earth. Welcome to this wonderful journey!

CHAPTER 1

Growing up

I was born in Amos, Quebec, Canada, a small cold French town where the winters seem to never end. I remember as a child how much I loved to sit in the grass during the short summers and play with the earthworms living under the tree stumps. I would let ants and spiders crawl into my hands and onto my arms; I could spend hours observing them with fascination. Unfortunately, I also remember being taught to catch the "bad" insects and make them suffocate in a jar filled with powdered detergent. I wish the previous generation had known better. But instead, the previous generation was taught to pull the wings off the flies... wow, it is about time to speak up for our insect friends!

My mother Ginette is what we have always called an "old soul". She is a born therapist with an attentive ear for anyone to tell their problems to. She seems to truly have a word of wisdom for everybody. She makes everyone feel special and loved, from her closest friends and family to pure strangers. She showers every soul she meets with love. When we were growing up, she would read us books about spirituality, about the after and before life and would often talk to my brother, sister and me about how we chose her to be our mom. All her teachings were supported (and still are) by countless metaphysical books written by world renowned mediums, such as Doreen Virtue and Sylvia Brown. We learned that as souls living in the spirit world, we prepare for our next incarnation on Earth by making a life plan. This life plan includes the goals, the details of our incarnation on Earth (place of birth, parents, siblings and friends – note that we often come back with the same souls), and the life lessons that will allow us to grow, with a life purpose and mission. Once everything is in place, we sign our official life contract and our journey on Earth begins.

The tricky part is to remember all or any of this when we arrive on this side in a human body. Children are obviously the purest form of beings, still uncorrupted by the modern society that we live in. They tend to have the strongest connection with the Source and can remember about their lives in the spirit world as well as their previous incarnations. Many children see colors around people (the auric field) or else talk about their past lives openly. A client of mine shared with me how her son told her all about his previous life in China. He talked about it like a grown man. Many adults unfortunately suppress instead of encourage the sharing of this precious knowledge and children grow up losing these precious skills. Society takes them away from their inner intuition and sensibility to the celestial world and those interactions not only stop but become forever forgotten.

Children also seem to have the strongest intuition in knowing what the future holds or guessing the sex of their upcoming sibling. For example: when the wife of my co-worker, Jose, became pregnant, their three-year-old son never changed his mind about the fact that he was having a sister. My three-year-old niece, as do many children, has told her parents more than once about seeing "people" in the house when there was no one physically present. Animals are also extremely intuitive and often hiss or bark at spirits visiting. My close friend Diana has witnessed her own cat hiss at the wall of the living room while her friend's two-year-old daughter was pointing and saying that a man was standing there. Diana and her boyfriend have both felt the presence of this spirit touching them with his cold fingers more than once. They know that a man died in their house prior to their buying it and, evidently, he appears to have trouble letting go of the physical world and moving on.

I have no clear recollection of my early childhood, although my mother says I did speak about the colors that I saw around people for a while. Nevertheless, I grew up to be pretty much like every other teenager (or almost). The only meat eaten at home was chicken and seafood. Halloween at our house meant giving out healthy honey-sweetened treats to our friends. Our friends did love us but called us the "natural" family. I kept drawings made by a friend in seventh grade showing me holding a block of tofu in the air while shouting: "natural, natural"! Today I am very grateful for choosing my mother. However, back then, as a teenager needing to "fit in", confusion and embarrassment grew. I needed my friends' approval and was only wishing to be like everybody else, doing what others were doing, even though I recall not having interest in what they were doing. However, back then I was convinced that fitting in was more important than doing what you love.

When my parents divorced at the end of high school, an interesting phenomenon occurred. My sister became acutely ill with juvenile rheumatoid arthritis. My mother was then only beginning to study the relationship between the mind and the body. She has now successfully completed intense training in this field and has countless numbers of patients to prove the theories, including my sister and myself. Growing up, one of our favorite hobbies was to read books about disease processes and their emotional cause. The information in these books sure made a lot of sense for my sister who suffered from profound stress during the divorce, bottling up her emotions to spare her younger siblings the emotional trauma. Consequently, her physical body got severely hurt.

When the time came to make a career choice for college, there was only one obvious choice for me: veterinary school. I had worked for the past two summers at the Refuge Pageau, a wildlife refuge in my home town, and had always loved animals. The program at the University of Montreal accepts about thirty nineteen-year-old students every year; the other half of the class is composed of older students. Fortunately, I was accepted immediately into the program. Veterinary school was an interesting time for me. Peer pressure was still present and trying to build my self-confidence was still using up a lot of my energy. Veterinary school offered a blend of very cultivated people. A lot of them were older, spoke English and had traveled outside of the country. It was very destabilizing for a young girl who knew nothing of the world except her own little French town. I kept comparing myself, feeling both inadequate and extremely different, although everyone was nice to me and seemed to accept me.

One weekend, my dad invited me to go skiing. I did not particularly enjoy the sport, but skiing was a "cool" thing to do at the time so I went, thinking that it would fill my need to fit in, and therefore, I would feel good about myself. The day ended with a broken thumb and no "cool" story to tell my classmates about the fall. There was just an embarrassing little slip on the snow that snapped my finger bone in two so badly that I ended up needing surgery. Of course, these breaks never happen to your non-writing hand. I struggled for two months in a cast, having to do everything with my weak hand, including writing my final exams. A question soon kept coming to mind: do you ever get hurt doing something you love, something you are doing for the right reason? Today I can answer yes to this question because at another point in my life, I took a major fall rollerblading, a time when I was so happy, thinking about how I was finally getting ready to leave an uncomfortable situation. Rollerblading while waiting for the train, I felt so good, light and free like a bird. Unfortunately, my imaginary wings were unable to support me and I hit the pavement resulting in quite a catastrophe. However, with second degree burns all over my right thigh and knee, I discovered the wonderful healing properties of silver sulfazalazine cream. This is a remedy that I now use frequently on burn patients. Hence my belief: everything happens for a reason. It has become clear in my heart what the lesson related to my broken thumb was: I should only do things for the right reason, for me; because I enjoy it; because it makes me happy; and it does not matter what others think.

School was going well. I was passionate about what I was learning and it was now time for some hands-on experiences. Something strange was about to happen during one of my large animal rotations. It was a cold winter day and I went on a farm call with my teacher to care for a calf that was having diarrhea. I was making a mental list of the possible causes of the diarrhea: parasitic like cryptosporidium, bacterial like salmonella, viral like…, and we ended up giving the calf intravenous fluids, antibiotics and a de-wormer. It was now four o'clock in the afternoon, we were just getting ready to leave the farm and while rinsing our equipment with the cold water coming out of the hose I asked my teacher what pathogen he thought was causing the diarrhea. He nonchalantly (in my view) answered that it did not matter as we will prescribe the same treatment anyway. By experience, I now know that viral diarrhea must take its course while we support the body with intravenous fluids, and prevent secondary bacterial infection with antibiotics. For a young animal prone to getting intestinal parasites, we will administer a broad-spectrum de-wormer as well. So my teacher was right in his teachings: cover your bases since tests do not exist for every single bacteria, parasite or virus. However, back then, being the thorough, meticulous and

4

perfectionist student that I was, I felt deeply upset that he did not care about knowing the exact cause of the diarrhea. My body went into shock in some way because the following day, at about four o'clock in the afternoon, my hands broke out into a rash and became covered with welts. The following day, the same thing happened at the same time. Within a week, it would happen anytime of the day when my hands would get cold, like they did at the farm while my teacher and I were having the shocking conversation. Within less than a month, my hands would break out with every change of body temperature, hot or cold. From my hands, it spread to my feet, knees and shoulders. I would come out of the shower covered with welts. By the end of the year, I did not even dare to wear short sleeves or shorts anymore. It was clear that the emotional shock I had experienced that day at the farm had triggered this intense physical response. I tried my best to heal, realizing that I had overreacted.

Graduation was around the corner and opportunities for additional specialized training were surfacing. By then, I had already spent two summers learning English and had completed six months of externships in America's top veterinary schools. I welcomed the opportunity to complete a one-year internship in a large emergency and specialty hospital in Michigan. What does not kill you must make you stronger. I am a survivor.

The hospital hired six interns that year. The following year, they took eleven. This tells you how much work there was to do and how exhausted we were. Countless nights without sleep, working in the overfilled emergency room, days and nights, preparing for rounds and presentations... I learned that when your body is not built for night shifts, it is just impossible to turn it around and sleep during the day. Six months into the year, I had to fight a cold that came with every sleepless emergency rotation and my veterinary school skin rashes now appeared religiously at the end of each twelve-hour emergency shift. My whole body would be covered with welts. Tired, exhausted and stressed, shedding tears became the only way to relieve the pressure. But somehow along the way, I had become allergic to my tears! My eyelids would blow up like balloons, keeping my eyes completely shut. How awful! I could not even do the one thing in life that at least brings a person relief and comfort. Now I only wanted to cry more. It was about time for the year to be over as my body was

5

on overload (although I will always be so indebted for all the great teachings, on a personal and professional level).

At that time, I was also struggling with a long distance love relationship. Between the good of having a boyfriend's support over the phone, there were the never-see-them-coming blow outs that would shake me deeply into my soul. Should I stay, should I leave? Once again, my body spoke the loudest. A kiss on the cheek from this man now set my skin on fire and here we go again. My face would get covered with welts. I could not ignore this much longer, could I? The last extremely important life lesson learned that year came from the time I was forced to spend alone. Spending one year in Michigan, without family or friends, became the best teaching grounds for a very important life lesson: listen to yourself, do what you love, find your passion, build your confidence. Although extremely destabilizing at first, I began to quickly enjoy this: I can wear whatever I want, listen to whatever music I want, even cut my hair. There was no one there to make comments about my choices or to make me second guess myself. How powerful and freeing! Life became much easier after that point. The internship ended and so did the love relationship. Finally my body began to heal. It took nearly one year to be completely free from any breakouts.

CHAPTER 2

I believe in miracles

I met my husband under fortuitous circumstances. I had just moved to the East Coast, a half-hour drive outside of New York City, and was finally starting to pay off my student loans with my first real job. My career was going well. It felt good to finally have so much free time to enjoy life as opposed to having my head buried under a ton of books. I could finally sleep eight hours every night. This was paradise! I was back to being single and felt great about having regained my own power. Once again friendless, but this time with lessons learned, I felt ready to rejoin society. I had a deep conversation with my father at that time during which I happened to describe what my perfect boyfriend would be like: sexy, taller than me with muscled shoulders, a sensitive soul who loves animals but who also has a tough, manly side of protecting his lady, and an artist (a musician preferably) since I do have some aptitudes in that field and thought that another artist would help me develop this side of my personality. God forbid I would fall in love with someone else in the medical field. For me, that would not work.

Having played basketball all during my childhood, I was not able to keep it up during college. However to me, the perfect way to have fun while exercising would be through dancing. I remembered a childhood dream of mine of taking ballroom dance lessons. I have always wished that I could move gracefully on the dance floor wearing a beautiful dress. It was now time to get back into physical shape.

It took me a while to find a dance studio in the area but I finally did. During my search, I had also found a gym close by and was giving it thoughts of joining. I called both the gym and the dance studio. While I had to leave a message at the dance studio, they signed me up right away at the gym and gave me a free first week trial. That very next day I started working out at the gym. Although I have always found it frightening to explore a new environment, I adjusted quickly and especially enjoyed the Pilates and aerobic classes. I finally heard back from the dance studio a couple of days later and my first try-out dance lesson (also free) got scheduled for the following week. The trial week at the gym went by quickly and I developed a routine that pleased me. I felt comfortable enough continuing to work out there and decided not to pursue dancing. Just the thought of showing up to dance class without a partner embarrassed me. Furthermore, having to re-adjust again to a new environment scared me, now that I had finally gotten comfortable at the gym. I did not think I had enough energy to do it all over again. So I made my decision to stay at the gym.

A few days went by until my childhood dream came back to haunt me, begging me to go to the free dance lesson. I had developed a knot in my stomach, which I now call my inner voice. However, at the time, this was a new feeling in my body that I did not know how to tame yet. In spite of all my best efforts and logical arguments trying to convince myself not to go to the dance studio, the only way to get rid of the knot in my stomach and feel inner peace again would be to obey to these higher forces and go to the dance studio. When your brain wants one thing but your heart wants another, I have learned that listening to your heart, your inner voice, your gut feeling, is always the way to go. So I started getting mentally ready to confront all the happy couples at the dance studio, who had signed up for classes to have a good time. I prepared myself for their looks of pity when they would see me arriving alone. Worse case scenario, I can just run out and find refuge at the gym. They can all think I am a sad case of loneliness and I can move on to rebuild my newly acquired self-esteem. Alright, let's just get this embarrassment over with already. Conquering all my fears, I arrived at the dance studio. There was only one other student present for what was also his first dance lesson. I felt better already. My dance teacher was kind of cute, taller than me and apparently working out. His name was Dan. He had strong shoulders and comforting hands. I quickly started enjoying dancing with him much more than with the student. The teacher's dog and faithful companion would accompany him to the dance studio everyday and socialize with the staff and students. Her name was

Hayley. I swear she had smelled the veterinarian in me because I could tell I would have to work hard to gain her trust.

So there was my answer, let's dance! I called the gym to let them know that I would not be back and started getting ready for my next dance lesson. I was having so much fun that I signed up for their golden package, which included unlimited numbers of group classes during the week as well as one weekly private lesson with my teacher. Although I was having a lot of fun dancing and laughing with Dan, I was still deeply burned from my previous relationship, and therefore was not looking for anything to happen between us. I had accepted the fact that I would never find my soul mate in this world and I was comfortable with never getting married or having children. Dan did share once a painful ex-girlfriend story that showed that his heart was hurt too much for him to risk getting hurt again. That being said, dancing quickly became immense fun and getting ready for the lessons would consume more and more of my time. I would participate in all of the group lessons, pretty much every night of the week, and could not wait for my private lesson with Dan at the end of each week. After a month, my teacher was getting sexier by the minute and dancing the merengue had gotten really hot! Finally came the point of no return and the knot in my stomach reappeared. I could not believe I would have to take such a huge risk. How dare I risk losing my dance teacher and all the fun we were having? Losing my new passion would just be too devastating. On the other hand, I could possibly gain so much more: maybe a life partner, maybe a soul mate. Unbeknownst to me, Dan was going through the same mental battle but with the added pressure of risking loss of his job, as dating a student was completely forbidden. The moment of truth came after one of our private lessons. I could tell that Dan, being so professional, would not venture on this territory: I would have to be the one breaking the ice. The knot in my stomach had now spread to my throat and I knew that letting the words out had become an emergency. I wrote my phone number down and passed it across the table in his direction while casually inviting him to call me if he was interested in hanging out over the weekend. The words that came out of his mouth were like a knife cutting through my soul as I heard him say that he was not allowed to hang out with students outside of the dance studio. I thought I was going to faint. The awkwardness of

9

the situation was building fast and I felt so foolish for jeopardizing our dancing relationship. Feeling sad and defeated, I began pulling back the miserable piece of paper, when suddenly he took it from me and put it in his pocket, saying that he might be able to make an exception. Phew!!! A feeling of relief spread through my entire body with hopes that I did the right thing by taking the risk. Maybe he would be the one I have been looking for all my life, my soul mate, my best friend, the love of my life. On my ride home, I kept looking at my cell phone thinking he could be calling anytime. I knew that I would not sleep at all that night.

Dan called me the same night and we met right away. We spent the whole night talking and walking on the beach with Hayley. It felt so good; I felt at home with him. After that night, Hayley loved me and started following me everywhere at the dance studio, giving our secret away! A month later, we were shopping for an engagement ring in the Diamond District of New York City. Love speaks louder than anything else. I knew I was going to marry him. None of my logical arguments against marriage bore anymore weight. My co-workers voiced their concerns about the craziness of my situation. How could I marry someone that I have known for less than two months? I felt deep in my heart that the mistake would be not to marry him. I did not need an in-depth, rational analysis of how crazy this seemed from the outside. What if we had known each other from a previous life and we were finally reunited? This is how I felt towards him.

Nevertheless, I caught myself a few times having moments of self-doubts where my brain would take over and try to convince me that I was crazy for wanting to marry him so soon. What do I do, listen to my head or my heart? How can you make the right decision when so madly in love? I had not shared any of this with my mother for fear of the emotional shock it would cause her. However, during a random conversation, she told me how she had recently met with a medium friend of hers. This sounded like the perfect idea for me. I had met with a medium once before and was truly intrigued by her abilities to know so many personal details about me. I deeply needed someone like that to restore some sanity in my life. I swore to myself I would not say anything about marriage to her. She did ask me to bring pictures of people close to me, and therefore, I brought one of Dan. She took a look at him and told me everything I needed to hear.

She gave me her approval and I ran out of her house with the most gigantic smile on my face. My mother figured out right away that there was going to be a wedding. The best thing was that she could only be supportive of it, since she had herself led the path to this. The visit with the medium did help her push all her worries aside. We had nothing left to do but celebrate this new love of ours.

A few incidents have since happened to strengthen my faith in the invisible world. One of them happened during the trip from New York to my home town in Quebec, where we were to be wed the next week. While driving through a national park, we hit a moose that was standing in the middle of the road, most likely trying to escape the heavy infestation of mosquitoes in the forest at that time of the year. Unfortunately, every year at this same location people die due to moose and vehicle collisions. When our vehicle struck the moose, the passenger side (my side) took the hit and the side window got completely shattered. I was not hurt, though. About a half hour before the accident, my extreme fatigue and discomfort in the front seat compelled me to go in the back of the van to sleep with Hayley in her doggy bed. I woke up in a frenzy to Dan zigzagging in the road trying to avoid the poor moose that was also running in all directions. That night, we both felt the Angels watching over us. We realized how deeply we loved each other and how much we wanted to spend our lives together. Dan was truly the perfect man for me, the one I had described to my father a few months before.

Dan was indeed a musician. One of high caliber, a rocker, with the most sensitive soul as well as a love and understanding of animals greater than anyone I have ever met. One of Dan's pets was a frightened but adorable silver Himalayan named Munchie. She had been abused, declawed and rescued several times until Dan finally gave her a stable and healing home. During this time, I had met a very sweet cat named Meeko at the veterinary hospital where I worked, who had been relinquished by a family that was unable to care for him. Meeko became our hospital cat until we could find him a good home. Having talked to Dan about him, we decided to take him home for the weekend with hopes of adopting him. Unfortunately, our poor friend Munchie got so scared and traumatized by his presence that she immediately started vomiting and having bloody diarrhea. We realized how stressful Meeko's visit was for her and returned Meeko to the hospital right away. Five days later, Munchie was still not back to her normal self and her health was continuing to decline. I tried everything the medical world had to offer without success. With embarrassment and guilt, I apologized to Dan for upsetting his feline companion and shared my worries of her never healing from this terrible experience. I fell asleep crying that night over him losing his dear friend Munchie. The following day, I woke up to a purring Munchie who seemed much brighter and even eating. What in the world happened? Dan confided that he had had a long talk with Munchie the night before and had told her how much we were sorry and how much we wanted her to stay with us and get better. She had nothing to fear as Meeko was gone and would never come back. I could not believe my ears or my eyes! Munchie was back to her normal self within just a few hours of this powerful talk. My mind could only continue to shift further away from the conventional medical teachings into the energy world and unexplainable extra powers that exist among us. I could feel my body becoming more attuned to these higher and more subtle vibrations. That was eight years ago. Munchie is well into her senior years today and is doing wonderful!

Life on the East Coast became quickly stressful with the constant traffic, high housing prices, lack of land, as well as gloomy and depressing winters. We began our quest to find a better world. We had a blast honeymooning in Florida. However, a move to Florida became rapidly out of the question due to the dreaded Hurricane season. California was at the top of our list, but we found it had the same familiar problems of traffic, crowds and high prices. However, it led us to Arizona. The majestic saguaros were impressive and won our hearts. Plus, Hayley would get to live on a lot of acreage, in a gigantic park, her favorite place! This was the most wonderful gift we could give her. We packed our modest belongings, along with Munchie, Hayley and our friend Hammy the hamster, and journeyed on a four-day drive to our new home with over five acres of land where the sun is always shining. I suddenly developed a sharp pain in the arch of one of my feet that lasted three weeks. The most plausible theory to this day remains emotional. Feet are the part of our body that helps us move forward. With the anxiety of a new move, my body followed my mind causing the pain in my foot. It took about three weeks to adjust to our new and better life. My foot healed during that time.

CHAPTER 3

Home euthanasia service for pets

In July of 2007, Hayley was fourteen years old and her breathing had slowly but progressively become labored, especially with exercise. She had also become incontinent and would urinate in the house. Considering her large size and age (which translates to being close to one hundred years old in human years), we were aware of our limited time left with her and focused on giving her as much quality of life as possible. After discussing our medical options and the risks of making her feel worse prematurely, we opted to not intervene but cherish each day with her.

One morning when I took Hayley outside to use the bathroom, I saw that something was wrong. Her breathing had worsened drastically and just a short walk sent her into a crisis where she could no longer catch her breath. Suffocating caused her to almost vomit. By some miracle, we managed to return into the house where she finally calmed down and returned to her normal self. Alarmed, I discussed the situation with my husband. We agreed that in order not to push her to that place of breathlessness again, we had to keep her extremely calm. We called Hayley's grandmother who had been a huge part of her life to get her input. She helped us make peace with the decision of helping her pass with dignity and not letting her suffer. We agreed to help her transition that night. Hayley had a great last day, comfortable in the air conditioned house in the company of Dan who had saved her life over twelve years before. I brought the necessary medications home from the hospital that night and a great friend and co-worker, Lisa, agreed to come help us and help Hayley have a peaceful passing in the comfort of home.

What we did seemed so surreal. After all these years of having Hayley around, how could we ever get used to her no longer being present? Were we ever going to be able to laugh and enjoy life again without her? I believed in life after death but I had never had any encounters with the spirit world.

Only a few months after Hayley transitioned into the next world, a canine named Moses became in need of the same help. Moses was Kristy's dearest companion and Kristy was Lisa's good friend. Kristy and I met for the first time when Lisa and I helped Moses transition in the comfort of home. Saying goodbye to a dear friend is, without a doubt, one of the hardest things to have to go through in life. Doing this in the comfort of home definitely brings peace to the whole family. Having experienced it myself, I deeply understand what other people go through when they have to make the decision to say goodbye.

I started thinking to myself, maybe I could offer this service to as many pets and their families as possible. How wonderful would it be if all pets could have a peaceful passing, with dignity, in the comfort of home? However, it would be scary to be on my own. Until then I had only been an employee. Owning my own business would require doing so much paperwork, licenses, where to start? What if things do not go well, I would not have another doctor to help me. The anxiety started building fast and I decided not to go through with this. A few days later the idea resurfaced. Although excited about how much good I could be doing, the more I thought about the amount of responsibility that would come with it, the more overwhelmed I became. I brushed off the idea many times and every time life would bring me back to it, reminding me of how grateful we were for Hayley to have had such a peaceful passing.

A few weeks went by until one evening when I was outside in the yard enjoying the darkness of the night and the many stars shining. For the first time, I felt Hayley's presence, hugging me from Heaven. It felt so real that I started crying. It became clear that she had been the one present all along, guiding each of my steps, keeping me on the path of starting a home euthanasia service. I suddenly began remembering who I was and what I had agreed to accomplish while on Earth. It was clear that embarking on this new journey was part of my life mission and life contract. Fighting it was pointless. I knew I had to surrender to Hayley, so I did. I asked her to please guide me safely on this new journey.

Right away, I met with Lisa to share my ideas, in the hope that she would be able to provide me with her unconditional support once again. Lisa was so enthusiastic that I knew that there would be no turning back. She looked at me and said, as if she was reading right off our souls' contracts, "The service should be called Hayley's Angels". The heavenly experiences I am about to share with you are truly priceless. My gratitude is endless toward Hayley and Dan, Lisa, Moses and Kristy, and all the pets and people who have crossed my path since, as I am a much better person today than I was before the birth of *Hayley's Angels*. Tapping into our own deepest potential and expressing it to its fullest is the most rewarding experience ever on Earth. Be the best you can be! Unleash your potential! Discover who you truly are!

Working hard on getting the service started, I knew the colors of *Hayley's Angels* would be fuchsia pink and white. Lisa finally found the perfect digital pink that would match my vision. Lisa contributed greatly in the creation of the logo, which was later perfected by Kristy and her husband Dave. I did not understand the reason for my sudden attraction to pink until later when I read in one of Doreen Virtue's books that pink is the color of love and compassion but also of protection while helping others. White being the ultimate color of protection, it however prevents from communicating adequately with the outside world. When your work involves supporting other people emotionally, pink is definitely needed to be able to give while protecting yourself and preserving your own vital energy.

I also quickly felt the need to have my clients address me by my first name instead of Doctor. Every time someone called me Doctor I would feel a wall building up between us. When people call me Joanne, I can feel a deep connection to them, on a human level and even more, on a soul level. I can feel this divine communion of souls helping another soul transition into the spirit world. This energy is so powerful that I can tell everyone in the room experiences the magic of the moment. It feels as we are touching Heaven and that I am fulfilling my life's purpose. Before leaving each home, I give everyone present a heartfelt hug as well. I truly feel that this is one of the most important moments of the procedure as love is truly the best healer.

I rapidly started feeling the differences in energies of the homes and people I would meet. Some are heavy, filled with pain, sadness and loneliness, whereas some are light, filled with happiness and love. Since I routinely transport the animals' bodies for cremation, I have noticed that pets themselves carry different energies as well, mostly always in tune with their family's energies. I had to learn to protect myself and cleanse my energy field to be able to help many families without feeling emotionally and physically drained. I routinely visualize myself in a bubble of protective white light and additionally ask my guardian Angels for maximal protection in times of increased vulnerability. I cleanse my chakras and aura regularly with a selenite crystal as well as with different visualization exercises, including one where a white shower of light is pouring over my head and whole body, removing any attached negative energy.

It hurts to lose a beloved pet, especially when we have to make the decision to let go. But that last act of friendship is the most loving and caring thing we can do for our best friend when our loved one is suffering and treatment is impossible. Allowing him/her to pass peacefully, with dignity, surrounded by family in the comfort of home, is the most extraordinary gift we can give him/her. Pets, like humans, do grieve the loss of a companion. This grieving process can be eased greatly by allowing pets to be present to say goodbye to their friend. Assisting to the procedure brings them closure and helps them recover faster. In-home euthanasia allows us to care for the whole family, two and four-legged members. My hope is that every sick soul on the planet gets to experience a peaceful passing, with dignity, in the comfort of home. I am hoping in writing this book to awaken everyone to the benefits of in-home euthanasia, for their loved ones and for themselves.

Knowing when it is the right time can be perplexing and making an appointment giving much time notice is often difficult. For most people, like me, once the decision is made, it must happen the same day. Emergencies often arise as well, and therefore, flexibility of the medical team is imperative in providing this service.

Please ask yourself these questions to assess your pet's quality of life: Is my pet in pain? Is my pet eating and drinking normally? Is my pet able to go to the bathroom without soiling him/herself? Is my pet doing his/her favorite things as he/she used to? Does my pet still have enthusiasm and interest for favorite toys, treats and family members? Is my pet able to go on walks, get up without assistance? Is my pet having more bad days than good days? Is my pet trying to tell me: "I need your help, it's time, I can't do this any longer" OR "I'm ok, I'd like to stay a little longer"?

Most important is, for everyone in the family, to feel at peace with the decision. This is imperative in order to be able to move on afterwards and to avoid second thoughts or feelings of guilt and regrets. Consult with your veterinarian. Perform all diagnostic tests needed to get answers that will help you make your decision. Remember that although the opinion of somebody you trust may be helpful, it may also bring more confusion. Trust your heart and your inner feelings. You know your pet best. Take it one day at a time.

If you are giving someone else advice for their pet, beware. Remember that since you do not live at their home nor see the pet every minute of the day and night, you will never get the complete picture of the situation. Listen to your friend or client's concerns and put yourself in his shoes. I feel the need to explain this concept as it can easily be misinterpreted. It is important not to put your own self in your friend or client's shoes. Instead, think of what you would do if you were him, with his abilities, his personality, his bond with his pet, his current situation and his life story. This is the best way to help him make the best decision, because you, yourself, may make a very different decision based on your different personality, different financial situation as well as different emotional state. Respect and support your friend's needs. Ask him to tell you how his heart feels. Remember that each pet, like people, comes into someone's life for a reason, to fulfill a specific mission. Some pets help us overcome a divorce, heal from a severe illness or are present through the loss of a family member or another difficult time in our lives. I helped a young couple's dog transition the day after their first newborn arrived. Lucky had been battling cancer but was doing fairly well until that day. It was truly as if he were saying, "My work here is done, now you have a new soul to care for, I can finally transition and relax." His physical body followed his mind in letting go.

I will always remember one of the strongest teams I have ever met: a feline named Poncho, who had been hit by a car and was paralyzed in his hind legs, and his human dad, who had also been traumatized and had trouble walking. Poncho could not defecate on his own because of the paralysis so dad had been physically assisting him for a couple of years, even administering stool softeners, which helped tremendously. While several people might have euthanized Poncho, his dad saw him as a wonderful supporter of his own condition: they both had physical handicaps, yet they both felt loved, accepted and "normal" together. Poncho and dad are a powerful team working at healing each other.

Many people also tell me how their pet told them when it was time to help them, giving them a clear sign. More and more people I meet are learning to listen to their inner voice and listen to their pets to know when to make this decision. Many people are afraid to share these "signs of guidance" with their family and friends by fear of being called crazy or laughed at. It can often be difficult for outsiders to recognize these subtle signs since they do not have the same emotional bond that the owner has with his pet. However, when you encourage someone to share how they truly feel, the answers become clear. Learning to sort out our feelings is extremely powerful in making the right decision as well: what do I want for myself, what does my loved one want and need? Being selfless is not easy, but is mandatory as our loved one's needs must precede our needs.

An example of this selflessness is the team of Tom and his dog, Sam. A few months ago, Tom called me to help him and his friend Sam, a handsome four-year-old Labrador retriever. Sam was battling cancer and his breathing had become extremely difficult. Tom knew it was time for his best friend to leave his physical body, and therefore, I was on my way to help them. Tom called me back a few minutes later telling me how he had to wait since his wife was out of town for another day and he felt guilty not to allow her to be present. I could feel the struggle he was going through. Knowing his wife personally, I began feeling the same struggle. Once I arrived, I could see how Sam's breathing was very rapid and labored. Could he last one more day? It was impossible to say for sure. He could deteriorate any minute and die suffocating. Natural death is not always peaceful. I have learned that some pets sacrifice themselves for their loved ones and are just not able to let go on their own. Sam seemed to be one of them: an extremely loyal friend who was particularly attached to his dad and so eager to please at all times that I could foresee a very unpleasant natural death, which was the last thing Tom wanted for his best friend. Sorting out our feelings, Tom and I agreed that Sam was ready and that keeping him one more day was not going to benefit him, his quality of live being already poor, it could only worsen. Tom finally looked at me and said, "I don't want to do this but I know in my heart it is time. Sam told me. He gave me the look earlier, asking for my help. My wife will have to understand." And of course she did.

Some dog breeds, for example, Chow Chow and German shepherd, are often so dedicated in protecting their families that quitting the "job" is out of the question. They keep on trying with all their might to be the good and young dogs they once were. These dogs need our help in freeing them from their physical bodies. I have learned the power of the mind from a few pets that I have found in horrific conditions. These pets were comatose, febrile, suffering with severely infected bed sores all over their bodies secondary to their inability to move in so long, dehydrated and emaciated secondary to starvation, yet they were not able to break the emotional ties and pass away on their own.

I remember one dog, Roxy. I had given her the usual sedative, which she took very well and fell asleep. Most pets, once the euthanasia solution travels through their body, stop breathing peacefully and transition, except for Roxy. Her breathing became rapid and her emotional struggle was evident. I told her to leave, that she was safe and that she was going to be able to continue watching over mom from Heaven. I told her that everything was going to be okay, that she was allowed to go and feel better. Nothing would help. I asked mom to give her permission to go. As soon as mom said the words, Roxy stopped her distressed breathing and left her physical body.

I often tell people who are struggling with their decision to have "the talk" with their four-legged friend. Allow him/her to go when the time has come. Pets do struggle leaving us as well. Tell your pet that you wish he would stay with you for many more years but leave it up to him. As hard as it will be to be separated for a while, he has to do what is best for him and go back Home when Home is calling. Thank him for all the good times together. He has been such a sweet companion and you will always love him. Somewhere inside, I think that everybody has the ability to transition peacefully and naturally once their life mission is completed, by sorting out their emotions adequately. Giving permission to our loved ones to follow their life plan and leave us when their time has come is extremely powerful in facilitating their transition. One of my clients shared with me how only a few minutes after she gave her own mother permission to leave, her mother transitioned peacefully.

I have helped a very sick dog whose owner was terminally ill as well. I felt so sorry for the suffering woman watching me free her friend and meanwhile, she had to continue suffering herself, now with the added pain of losing her loyal companion. While giving Angel her injection, I asked her to help mom from Heaven and heal her from her suffering. Two days following Angel's transition, mom was able to free herself and join Angel in Heaven. They had truly helped each other.

I have encountered so many situations where people tell me how their pet got better right after we talked on the phone as if they heard us and do not want to leave yet. I do believe pets feel the energy around them. When this happens we certainly cancel the appointment immediately. The opposite happens as well. Some pets start deteriorating rapidly after the phone call as they finally feel allowed to go. They feel their family accepting their departure and giving them permission to leave, therefore, they stop fighting and sacrificing themselves for their loved ones. This brings the family comfort in seeing that they made the right decision. In those instances, I do not always have time to arrive at the home before the pet has already transitioned.

Here is the story of Roux. She was a fifteen-year-old feline who had been vomiting for weeks, was becoming lethargic and had lost weight in spite of a fairly decent appetite according to her owner over the phone. She was one of those cats that get extremely stressed leaving the house. Roux was a rescued cat whose previous owners had allowed outside, where she had become injured. They took her to the shelter in the hope that she would get adopted. The shelter staff was unable to medicate her, or even touch her, and felt she would have to be euthanized. That was when her current owner found her. Eleven years later, mom knew she would be unable to take Roux to the veterinary hospital without causing her great distress. At her age, there were a few metabolic diseases that could be causing her symptoms. I could tell how difficult it was for mom to make the decision to let her go. Between two episodes of sorrowing and shedding tears, we managed to tentatively schedule a time to meet the following day. Mom said she would call to confirm in the morning. The next morning, I received her phone call and prepared to meet with her in the afternoon.

When I saw Roux, I was extremely surprised by how good she looked. She seemed to have quite a bit of energy and a decent weight. She also ate eagerly the treats that I had brought over without vomiting. I started thinking to myself: can I really euthanize her? Maybe she has only a minor ailment that can be cured. How can I question the owner's motives and more than anything else, how do I discuss with her my doubts after I saw how upset she was and still is today? I do not want to torture her any further especially since Roux might be hiding a more serious illness. Considering that mom can not medicate her either, I would hate to have to euthanize her anyway after causing both her and mom so much more stress, I would feel guilty for the rest of my life. I need emergency guidance from the Universe. As I was struggling with my thoughts, mom said, "She slept with me last night, which she had not done in quite some time. It was her way of telling me that she approves of my decision. She knows what is going on."

I instantly felt better and at peace with Roux's soul purpose and my own role to play in the process. I was sent into their lives to bring them unconditional love and support. I must trust the Universe that this is the right decision for this family. I must accept not knowing if I could have saved her. I then realized that what mattered most was how we felt about the situation. Mom felt at peace, I felt at peace. We therefore proceeded in helping Roux transition. As I was getting ready to leave their home, mom approached me with a very special gift to show her immense gratitude. She handed me a heart-shaped rose quartz crystal and told me its meaning: my unconditional love and compassion shown towards them. She thanked me deeply for helping her and Roux!

This meaningful gift confirmed that I had completed my mission successfully and fulfilled my purpose with this family. I could not have been happier. Mom felt at peace, supported and approved of, which allowed her to find closure. The process was peaceful for her and her feline friend. To this day, Roux's heart follows me everywhere I go. I hold it tight against my heart when I need guidance and strength in helping others. This powerful experience taught me that life is truly about perception. What matters is how you feel and how you make others feel. Whatever combination of actions and decisions that brings peace inside is the right way. Someone else in this situation might have taken Roux to the hospital for diagnostics, or might have wanted to sedate her at home to perform blood tests, or might have felt differently about the meaning of Roux sleeping with mom. But Roux had been sent into mom's life for a reason. Outsiders can not question someone's feelings as only this person's feelings can decide the meaning of a sign as well as the rightness of an action that follows.

CHAPTER 4

Encounters with the spirit world

"Smile when you think of me, Because I do when I think of you"

Animals, like people, have emotions. They also have a soul and we all go to the same place after leaving our physical bodies. The death of the physical body represents the freeing and transitioning of the soul from the Earthly plane into Heaven, also called Home. Although I have always believed it, Hayley gave me the confirmation after she transitioned. Ninety-nine percent of the families I help share these beliefs as well, which also in most instances have come from powerful life experiences. My friend Louise is convinced that she visited Heaven during her surgery. Over there, she was offered the option of coming back into her physical body or not. She chose to return by the side of her husband. Another friend, Bob, during a severe illness that led to loss of consciousness, also visited Heaven but was instructed to come back to Earth to continue his life mission.

I believe that each life is meaningful, unique and special. Each life counts and each transition to Heaven should be done in a respectful manner during a divine moment. Max's family told me that a few minutes following his transition, as I was driving away from their home, everyone saw a clear dog head-shaped cloud in the sky that looked just like Max. Mom's faith had been shaken and put to the test during the few weeks preceding Max's transition. Mom was let down by two close friends telling her that dogs do not go to Heaven. Although hurt by those comments, mom continued to believe and any remaining doubts completely disappeared when Max signaled at them from the sky, confirming that indeed, all dogs go to Heaven!

A good client and friend of mine, Ann, also confided how following the loss of her father she recognized his face in the clouds as well. She was even able to photograph it. When I saw his picture next to his cloud picture, I was speechless as it was identical!

I have witnessed other examples of animals signaling their arrival in the spirit world. Boullie was Mary's very wise canine teacher and guide here on Earth. As soon as I met him to help him in his transition, I felt his powerful energy even though it was night time and we were outside in the dark. Immediately after his spirit left his body, all the dogs in the neighborhood started howling in unison, welcoming Boullie to the other side. A similar situation occurred when we went to the park to assist Violet in her transition. Violet was a very old kitty who loved grass. During our ceremony, I noticed a handful of geese getting closer to us. As soon as Violet left her physical body, they all started chanting what we now call "The Goose Song!"

So many clients have told me about how their pets grieved the loss of their companion. Although some pets do celebrate the increase in attention given to them, some others become completely lost. In all cases the dynamic changes. I have come to realize that the intensity of the grieving process depends largely upon the relationship among the pets as well as the opportunity they have to obtain closure. For example, if the alpha pet transitions, it is much harder for his followers to cope with the loss of their leader. On the other hand, an independent and self-confident pet will adapt much more easily to the loss of a subordinate. The eternally young souls, who always want to play because they only see the bright side of life, do adapt easily to the loss of a companion. Pets that are extremely people oriented will celebrate the departure of their competitor as they will receive more attention. For most animals, being present during the transition of their housemate is extremely beneficial as it brings them understanding and closure. I always encourage families to allow every member of the pack to be present. Dogs and cats usually join proportionately to their needs. Some prefer to watch from a distance, while some others, including my friend Tater Tot the bunny, needed to be right next to his sick friend as the official moral supporter. I see how beneficial this can be for the dying pet as well. Again, based on their personality, some sick animals need as much support as they can, whereas others so desperately want to be alone that they end up transitioning when no one else is home. If the decision is made to separate pets during the euthanasia process, I think allowing everyone to visit with the deceased body is extremely powerful in bringing closure and understanding as well.

The loss of a true sibling or a close friend can lead the lonely pet to severe illness and even death himself. For that reason, I have on a few occasions helped two pets transition together. I will always remember the beautiful story of Beethoven and Savannah. These two siblings spent their whole lives together minus one day. They loved each other and did everything together. The day that Savannah got sick and had to stay one night at the hospital, Beethoven became so depressed that their family decided never to separate them again. By the age of fourteen, their health had significantly declined as they were blind, deaf, arthritic and diabetic. It was time to help them transition. It was so comforting to be able to do this for them. Among the tears, everyone was smiling and wishing to have a twin to share life with as well as death. Beethoven and Savannah's bodies were positioned next to one another, hugging, and were cremated together.

Let me share the story of a bully cat named Samantha. Samantha had lived with three other cats for many years. Samantha was ruling the house and keeping her three subordinates confined in one bedroom. One evening, her family came home and found that Samantha had pushed the window screen open, allowing everyone to get outside and was guarding the window so no one could come back in. When her turn came to transition, no other cat was around to be seen. As soon as her soul left her body, the three other cats came out of the bedroom to celebrate, rubbing everywhere and purring. Their relief and approval of the departure of Bully Samantha was obvious.

When Misty passed, her boyfriend Bear lay in her grave for an hour. Cowboy visited his best friend's grave site for a week. Their families did the right thing by allowing them to do so and get the closure they needed. These experiences make me strongly believe that all pets should transition from the comfort of home for their benefit as well as the benefit of all family members. In the instance that a sick pet is already in the hospital and performing the euthanasia on site eases the stress on the animal, I suggest that the other pets be allowed to visit their departed friend or else that the deceased pet be brought home to allow everyone to understand and find closure. I have heard too many stories of pets that do not know where their friend went, and therefore, spend hours waiting at the door or looking for them. They stop eating, are restless, depressed, may do a lot of sighing or have trouble sleeping. Grieving pets can show many symptoms identical to those experienced by the bereaved pet owner.

The same concept applies when the animal's master dies. In most instances, people transition in the hospital and pets never understand what happened to their master as they never see them come home. A widow's story was published in the newspaper when her husband died and his dog never got to say goodbye. For one week following his death, his dog did not eat and waited at the door for him to return. Finally, the widow, out of desperation, took her dog to the cemetery. The dog right away found his master's grave and lay down for several hours. When he was ready, he returned home and was finally able to move on and return to his routine.

Should children be present during their pet's transition? I have found that age does not matter as much as personality. Everyone has unique needs. Whereas some adults are emotionally unable to be present, some children are fascinated with the process. Children younger than three years of age do not usually understand much of what is happening, and therefore, do not seem to grieve much, especially if there are other pets living in the home to distract them. What is the last mental image that you want to keep? How would you like to be involved? Discussing with each family member what is going to happen is important. Everyone should feel comfortable assisting with the entire procedure, only part of it or not at all. Everyone should do what makes them feel the most at peace. The procedure can be done inside or outside the home, in the pet's favorite area. A sedative is first given to allow the pet to relax and fall asleep, peaceful and pain free. Once asleep, the euthanasia solution is given. Although it is never easy to say goodbye to a friend, the procedure is usually very peaceful to watch.

It is extremely healing for people to personalize their ceremony as much as possible. I always let the family decide if they and their pet would rather be inside or outside the house. The family also decides if they want to feed their pet something special. We fed Casey a mountain of cheese as she fell asleep while Sharky-Blue was fed chocolate-coated pretzels. I encourage families to take their pet for a last walk, feed a last burger or anything else their pet loved to do. I will always remember Belle and her ice cream and apple pie farewell party, with her human and animal friends. Everyone who knew and loved Belle gathered to share stories and pictures, to give her hugs, kisses and vanilla ice cream. One by one, Belle visited each guest, giving hugs, kisses and saying goodbye in her own sweet and graceful way. One ceremony that I also particularly enjoyed was during Buddy's transition. Dad would regularly share his beer with his best friend, therefore, we filled Buddy's dish with beer and she fell asleep while sharing a last drink with dad. Some people sing, play guitar or flute, play a pet's going-to-bed song that was part of the routine every night, give a massage, or watch the sunset. One dog licked his best friend's ears until he fell asleep. Between tears, we smile and laugh, remembering the fun times shared with the pet, the favorite things he used to do and that we will miss. I always love to learn how the family met with their pet in the first place. We talk to the pet, tell him how much we love him, thank him for all the good times, tell him to enjoy his new, young and healthy body in Heaven and that we know he will be watching over us. When a pet has a favorite location, I try to honor it even when it means crawling under the bed to help Molly transition peacefully and comfortably.

So many clients have shared with me stories of how their departed loved ones came to visit them from the spirit world, often in their dreams but also in scent and in sight. My friend Thomas and his brother regularly smell the cigar that their father used to smoke. They firmly believe that it is his way to let them know that he is visiting. A canine named Buddy rang the bell of his collar to cheer up mom. There is a great book written by Kim Sheridan called *Animals and the Afterlife* that I always recommend to my clients to validate what they are experiencing. When I helped the feline Bat Baby in her passing, her best friend, Toby, came up on the bed and fell asleep on this very book. When Molly's turn came to transition, mom asked me to come the very same day if possible. My schedule was full until nine o'clock in the evening. However, due to her location, I thought I would be able to make myself available at around seven o'clock. Molly's dad had transitioned just a few months before at the exact same time. Mom strongly felt that this was a sign from her husband telling us that he was present in welcoming Molly into Heaven. Mom also confided how her husband loved to play golf and since his transition, her family keeps finding golf balls at the least expected locations. They believe this is his way to tell them that he is watching over them. Another client confided that he and his family started seeing hummingbirds after their father transitioned, this bird being his favorite. His family is unanimous about believing that it is a sign from their father visiting. A friend's ill grandmother told her family that she was going to meet with her deceased husband the following day at five o'clock. The next day, she indeed transitioned into the next world just a few minutes before five o'clock.

I was driving home the day that a dear canine friend of mine, Papi, transitioned in the hospital. I suddenly felt his strong presence near me and I knew he had reached Heaven safely. Filled with sadness, I told him how much I loved him and that he had been such a sweet and handsome boy. I got the urge to turn on the radio, and when I did, the song playing was "I Give You the Best of My Love", by The Eagles. This song spoke strongly to me as if it were Papi's way to tell me that he loved me, too. Tears ran down my cheeks as I felt his heavenly love wrapping around me.

When Treva called me to help Jessie, I unfortunately was unavailable until the evening. Treva had talked to several veterinarians over the phone but since she connected best with me, she decided to wait for me. To confirm her decision, she picked an Angel card for me from a deck created by Doreen Virtue. The card read "Blessing". This consoled Treva in her feeling that it was the right thing to wait for me to help her and Jessie. That night, the Angels were waiting for us. When I entered her house, I felt the presence of several divine creatures that had joined us to guide Jessie in her transition. The room was filled with divine love that Treva and I both felt intensely. That night, we followed Jessie into Heaven. As Jessie's spirit transitioned from one world to the next, Treva and I experienced extreme peace. We felt wrapped in a blanket of heavenly love and hugged by the Angels. No words can come close to describing our state of supreme peace and communion with the celestial world. That night with Jessie, Treva and I definitely touched Heaven.

Here are some meaningful ways to honor a pet's memory. Most importantly, I always encourage families to continue talking to their pets even after they have left their physical bodies. Ask them for guidance and strength. It is also important to heal any unresolved emotion. Tell your pet everything you wish you had said to him and things you wish you had done differently. You can write a letter to express your feelings. Write a poem or story about your pet. Make a clay paw print or keep a lock of hair. Hold a memorial service or candle ceremony at home or in a place that was special to your pet. Arrange a designated shelf with framed photographs of your pet along with your pet's favorite toys or belongings. Make an album of photographs, stories and poems written by family members that tell about cherished memories of your pet.

The death of a pet means the loss of a companionship, a non-judgmental love source that we used to care for and nurture. One needs to be patient with themselves or others experiencing loss. Studies have found that people often go through similar stages of grief although responses to loss can be as diverse as the people experiencing it. If you give yourself time, healing will occur. Acknowledge your grief and give yourself permission to express it. Cry as much as you need. Only YOU know what your pet meant to you. Get lots of rest, good nutrition, drink plenty of water and exercise. Surround yourself only with people who understand your loss. Do not be afraid to get help. Take advantage of support groups and grief counselors. Accept the feelings that come with grief. Talk, write, sing or draw. Indulge yourself in small pleasures. Be patient with yourself. Consult your own "Higher Power", either religious or spiritual.

CHAPTER 5

Caring for ALL animals

The beginning of 2009 marked a new chapter in my life as I woke up from the modern materialistic society that I grew up in: a society of consumption, destruction and pollution where most people's primary focus is themselves supported by the belief that money rules all. The biggest revelation came regarding my diet. I could suddenly feel the pain of all the animals that I had been eating. The more I learned about the horrible lives these animals endured before ending up on my plate, the more disgusted I became. The more I read about wildlife habitats and oceans being destroyed, the more ashamed I felt to be a part of the so-called superior human race. Words and images of what I had discovered kept racing in my head: "Time is money, the industry doesn't have time to care;" sows and dairy cows separated from their babies; laboratory mice suffering from Botox. Industry animals are the biggest polluter of our waterways and the biggest consumers of water; the meat industry causes more global warming than all cars, boats and planes together; converting plant protein into animal protein is wasteful and counterproductive; shrimp fishing is the most environmentally destructive practice.

It was time to make one of the most important decisions of my life: I was not going to participate in the destruction of my planet. I love and care for all living creatures, therefore, I want them to have the good life they deserve: all creatures, great and small, have equal footing in the circle of life. Every creature is unique, special and important for our world's balance. Everyone has a reason for existing. Teamwork makes life easier for everyone and I wanted to be a part of the team. That is why I became vegan. Veganism is defined as living without exploiting animals, therefore eliminating the use of animal products for any purpose: in the diet, including eggs and dairy products, as well as in cosmetics, medications, leather goods and more. My own definition of veganism extends to eliminating from my lifestyle all products tested on animals or made by harming animals in any way. Adopting a green lifestyle is therefore closely connected. Caring for the planet means caring for animals including recycling to save trees and resources, using electric cars or carpooling for cleaner air, collecting rain water and preserving water, developing and growing renewable and sustainable resources such as bamboo, lyptus and hemp to make clothes, furniture and oil, and maximizing wind and solar energy.

Suddenly Dan and I realized how sad the world we lived in was, and that a vegan lifestyle could improve it. The arguments for choosing a vegan lifestyle include: all industry animals could be pets and should be treated like pets; the relationship between a mother and her baby is sacred and must be protected to preserve the mental and physical health of both beings, through love, safety and guidance; eighty percent of agricultural land in the United States is used to grow food to meet the needs of factory-farmed animals; twenty vegetarians could be fed on the amount of land used to feed one meat-eater; animal proteins cost five times more than plant proteins; vegetarian and vegan are healthier as they have lower rates of cancer, hypertension, diabetes, obesity and heart disease; cotton is a water-intensive crop and heavily fertilized; it takes 2900 gallons of water to produce one pair of blue jeans; 816 600 gallons are used during the life of one cow; it takes 1857 gallons of water to produce one pound of beef; if everyone decreased by ten percent their meat consumption, it would free over twelve million grains annually to feed the planet. To sum up: adopting a vegan lifestyle (eating plant protein) stops animal cruelty, saves money, helps the environment, decreases pollution and global warming, preserves water, stops world hunger, makes you healthier and happier to be contributing in a huge way to healing your world.

Dan and I immediately started reusing our shopping bags and became aware of the impact on our world with every action we took. Little by little, we found cruelty-free shampoo and soap, new laundry detergent and cleaning products, new ways to live in harmony with our world. Since fish living in contaminated waters accumulate heavy metals, we started getting our daily ration of essential fatty acids in seaweed and algae oil vegan capsules (Flora

DHA vegetarian algae). Dan created a small appliance and electronic recycling service to encourage repairing and reusing as opposed to trashing and consuming. I began reading every label on every product at the store (and called some companies to clarify their authenticity), started shopping regularly at health food stores, and became familiar with the vegan logos on the animal friendly products. I read books about veganism and how to eat healthier. I have removed as many preservatives, chemicals, pesticides, genetically modified organisms, processed and artificial foods from my diet as possible. I try to eat products that are as close to nature as possible: fresh, raw and organic fruits and vegetables as opposed to cooked (which decreases the nutritional value) along with legumes, sprouts and whole grains. I started feeling so much better in my skin and found a new energy as well: no more wanting to nap after a large, fatty meal. It did not take long for my body to adjust positively to this new way of life. The change was so drastic that on the few occasions where I had to eat non-vegan food, I could now taste their preservatives. My body could never go back to artificial meals that I used to eat. My research extended to the pet food industry as well, to find the few diets offering free range meat, dehydrated or freeze dried as opposed to cooked, preservative free and organic. I realized also that one does not need much food or resources to survive. Everyone should be very careful of wasting even the smallest thing. If you consume dairy products or meat, find the farms who care about their animals and who provide them with a true free range environment. Support the happy farms that raise happy animals, that give them good lives and a quick, painless and dignified death. Animals should die for our survival only. Be respectful, responsible, grateful, and say "thank you" to the animals sacrificing their lives for you.

Besides using animals for food, I believe there are a few other "society-approved" but animal cruelty-filled practices. Greyhound racing and other gambling sports focus more on the money aspect than on the animals' well-being. Catch-and-release fishing should also be stopped since nearly fifty percent of the fish will die due to the stress and injuries of the capture, while the other half of the fish remain alive and suffer from their injuries. What about rodeos? Are rodeos kind to animals? What if this were done to you? How would you feel? Is this all necessary? Is this for our pleasure or our survival? It is time to question the system in place and our society's standards.

I also find it necessary to mention that if an animal gets killed for any reason, road accident for example, we should most definitely make the best use of its body by recycling and not wasting. I will always admire my Chinese roommate from the East Coast for following her cultural tradition to eat and utilize as many parts of the animals as possible. Even though it was hard to watch her slice the pork kidneys and prepare the chicken feet for the stew, I wish everybody could be as mindful as she is. Along the same lines, Dan and I plan on rescuing a few chickens in the future for a couple of reasons. First, chickens make wonderful pets as they can be readily trained, much like a dog. In fact, according to the literature, chickens are smarter than dogs. I would love to have a chicken friend sitting on my shoulder while going for a walk. Kathy, a client and friend of mine, has proven that chickens are indeed quite smart. She trained her chickens to run a mini-agility course, and they seemed to learn each obstacle more quickly than her dogs learned their agility obstacles! The second reason for rescuing hens is to utilize the eggs that they naturally provide. At our house, they will be showered with love, and therefore, will have the happy life they deserve.

During this period of shift in consciousness, I came home one night and found a praying mantis on the ramp of the staircase leading to the house. It was waiting on the very spot where I always put my hand. This poor creature had gotten trapped in a spider web and its feet were stuck together. I rapidly found a small twig to use as my surgical instrument and very carefully I separated its legs by removing as much web as I could. I felt so good about helping another creature in the circle of life. The praying mantis seemed to feel the love as it waited for me to be completely done before it freely hopped away. This experience sparked my return to a childhood passion: saving the insects. I became filled with peace to have finally come full circle and returned to the pure soul that I was as a child, loving all of nature's creatures, even the smallest. Since then, every time I find a drowning insect in the kitchen sink, I slide a fork underneath it and slide it onto a paper towel to dry. I have quickly become amazed at the number of presumed dead insects that only need a little help to get back on their feet. My experience has now shown that most insects drowning in the kitchen sink can be saved! For the undesirable insects flying in the house or crawling rapidly on the floor, I created "The Bug Saver", made of 100% recycled materials. Anyone can make one because it is made with common materials. To make one, take an empty cereal box and an old see-through plastic container that has lost its lid. Cut one of the largest sides of the cereal box into a piece big enough to cover the open end of the plastic container, and there it is! Cover the insect with the plastic container and slide the piece of cardboard underneath. Hold it all together tightly until you reach the outdoors to free your insect friend. If you feel the need to distance yourself from the insect, split the end of an empty paper towel roll and tape it to your plastic container as a handle. You will soon feel immense joy at giving someone its freedom as opposed to crushing it needlessly. Teach kindness to children, family members and friends by example. Inspire others!

One of the best books that I have read is called: *Eating in the Light*, again written by Doreen Virtue. It made me realize how being vegan goes hand in hand with being a cleaner channel of communication with the animals, the Universe and the spirit world. For the first time, the psychic realm and my vegan world were fusing and this was truly wonderful! It made a lot of sense as my body had already began to feel cleaner and more attuned with higher universal vibrations. As stated in the book, meat carries a heavier energy compared to live food like fresh fruits and vegetables. Meat also contains the energy and emotions of stress and pain of the animals that died. This was easy for me to relate to since I had already experienced the differences in energy of the euthanized animals I had helped.

I learned that another way to cleanse our body, mind and soul, and develop our psychic abilities is by decreasing our exposure to electromagnetic waves from sources such as televisions, computers and electronic devices. My body was already teaching me this lesson on its own by increasing my sensitivity to all electronics. I have come very close to fainting half a dozen times while being exposed to strong levels of electromagnetic waves. I now always try to use an ear piece when talking on the phone and restrict my time in front of the computer and television. I only watch uplifting programs since the ones that carry the heavy energy of anger, hate and fear, e.g., horror movies, damage the auric field. I had already instinctively stayed away from them for those exact reasons. The same goes for the people surrounding us: negative people do deplete us from our vital energy and act as a source of pollution. We should surround ourselves with people whose energy flows harmoniously along with ours. Advertisements are also a powerful source of negative bombardment from society and should be avoided. As you become a cleaner channel of communication, your energy shifts and your sensitivity develops to a point where you can no longer tolerate food that you used to eat or activities that you used to do, like visiting noisy and crowded places or enjoying a fast and shaky carnival ride.

As an ultimate act of healing myself and contributing to healing my world, I felt the need to organize an annual *Caring for ALL Animals Celebration Day* in Tucson, Arizona. The event is held every November and this year 2011 marks our third annual event. My client, Connie, has been a huge supporter since the first day she heard me talk about it. She was blessed with a wonderful animal encounter shortly after the first event: she was taking a walk in the park when she found a baby raven that had fallen off the tree. On subsequent walks, she brought food to him and continued to feed him everyday until he was finally able to fly a few weeks later. This is when her baby raven decided to follow her all the way back home. Unfortunately, neighbors were inconvenienced by his presence and started throwing rocks until he finally flew away. Saddened, Connie visited the park a few weeks later. As she noticed a flock of ravens flying above her, one broke away and flew towards her. It was her baby greeting her to say, "Thank you for saving my life."

CHAPTER 6

Tapping into the power of our past lives and Animal Communication

I came to the realization a while back that our hospital work crew had become extremely fascinated by the invisible world. Several co-workers were comfortable sharing their special encounters and talking about them quickly became as normal as saying that we went to the movie or the mall over the weekend. We had all helped each other, and continue to, awaken our dormant potential. Reading the book *Earth Angels* by Doreen Virtue really answered some fundamental questions that I had about who I was and why I had always felt so differently from the people surrounding me, at all ages of my life. The book also spoke deeply to my husband (to his huge surprise!) and brought him inner peace and understanding of who he was on a soul level. There had always been more than meets the eye and this book confirmed it. Little by little, I realized how many friends and clients shared my ways of thinking and I found it wonderful to be able to grow with them in sharing our life experiences.

Approaching the end of the year 2009, the hot topic of discussion became past life regression. My friend Diana had participated in many sessions and had learned through them that her current abdominal problems were linked to a past life, where she was hurt in the stomach. Her body today was still suffering from it, referred to as cellular memory. I thought it was a fascinating concept and was interested in learning more about it.

Coincidentally, shortly after this conversation, I received an e-mail invitation to attend a past life regression workshop from Judy, an Energy worker. I had recently met Judy over lunch to discuss my home euthanasia service. The timing could not have been better for such an opportunity, therefore, I immediately signed up. This workshop enriched my life tremendously. It deepened my understanding of who I am on a soul level as well as answered some existential questions that I had had for many years. Judy guided us into a deep meditative state and visualization of past incarnations. The whole session was in fact pretty short but truly felt like a magnificent voyage throughout lifetimes (which it was). Traveling in a canoe down the river of my past lives, my first stop was as a fisherman. I saw myself wearing big boots and coverall, unloading my boat and transporting my daily catch to the market. I was the father of about eight children (there were too many to get an accurate count but the house seemed full!). I had a wife caring for them. My job was to provide for the whole family. I felt confident that with continuous hard work, one day at a time, we were going to be okay. I thought this life experience was probably responsible for my current faith in life that things will always work out, as long as we are dedicated and trying our best.

My second stop was on a sandy beach, with tall red mountains in the background, really similar to the ones found in the southwestern United States. Perhaps I have lived here before, hence my deep feeling of having returned home in this current life, in Arizona. What are you wearing? What do you see? Judy would guide us in looking around and describing the landscape, the clothes we were wearing... I saw myself as a Native American woman. It felt so familiar. My partner of life was a friend of mine in this current life. I died giving birth to our child. Wow, fascinating! This explains so much! I have a huge and unexplained fear of giving birth that even my mother can not explain. Here is finally a valid explanation for it.

Vincent and I grew up together (in this life time) just a few streets away from each other. Somehow, we ended up in the same class from kindergarten to fourth grade until my family moved across town and I changed schools. Vincent has always loved the outdoors and feels at home in the forest. He is the most caring hunter I know, living off the land, respecting the land like the great Indian Chiefs do. This past life regression explains so much of his behavior and personality today. When we were children, he would bring me gifts: feathers, bird wings and feet that I would put neatly in an album. Vincent's passion for the woods today, combined with his Indian lifestyle has even led him to lose his writing skills from not using a pen in over sixteen years. Needless to say, technology and computers mean nothing to him. Most people can not understand him, and neither could I, until now.

The other amazing discovery from the past life regression was the understanding of my relationship with Vincent in this life. I had never been able to explain why we had always felt so comfortable around each other, like we have known each other forever, in spite of the short time truly spent together in this current life. Our interactions currently occur about every ten years and each time, it feels like we just spoke the day before as we share the smallest slices of our lives, which we always find very funny. I feel truly blessed to be able to continue a relationship that started a lifetime ago!

I reunited with my current life's husband on my third stop during my past life regression. We lived together during medieval times. We appeared to be in our teens and true love was developing. The movie of our lives was short but intense: I saw myself racing up the tall flight of stairs in the castle, looking desperately for my soul mate, when suddenly I saw myself crumbling in sorrow as one of the castle knights announced that Dan had gone horseback riding in the forest and was killed. No chance to say goodbye? This was so impossible and unfair. I felt so alone. My love, the one I was going to marry, my best friend, got stolen from me forever.

Since the first day I met Dan in this current life, I have had the strangest feeling of needing to enjoy each day with him to the fullest because our time together may be short. This way of thinking was surprising to me and foreign to my given personality. I always wondered where it came from and am so grateful now to have found the answer.

The skills learned during this powerful experience prepared me for the next step in my life: Animal Communication. When Kristy, Lisa and I helped Moses transition in 2007, we were not aware of how deeply pets can grieve the loss of their companion. Kristy had made the decision to keep Nuru in the garage while Moses transitioned. None of us even thought of allowing Nuru to see his body so she could understand where he went and get closure. We all wish we could go back in time and fix our mistake.

Shortly after losing her leader, her protector and dear companion, Nuru developed severe eye problems, which she is still struggling with today. It took us a while to link the two together. Nevertheless, her problems led to Kristy and I having a conversation about emotions and physical diseases and how we both believed they were related in Nuru's case. Kristy decided to seek help from an animal communicator, who was able to tell us how difficult it had been emotionally for Nuru to cope with the loss of Moses. It had in fact been so difficult that her physical body was being severely impacted as well. Lee and Anna, close clients of mine, had used the services of an animal communicator as well in the past and were thrilled to share with me their experiences. Fascinated to learn more about this, I remembered Judy and contacted her to participate in her next animal communication classes.

Animal communication is accomplished in the same way mediums perform their work: via telepathy. Energy is unbounded by the constraints of time or space. By entering in communication with an animal's energies, we can learn more about an animal's likes and dislikes, emotional issues and medical problems. Healing can then start at an energy level. Animal communication helps animals share their point of view, is an opportunity for animals to express themselves and allows us to explain certain things to help them understand and heal behavioral as well as physical problems. Animal communication is a wonderful tool for elderly and/or ill pets to express how they want to be cared for, and treated or relieved from their suffering. They can tell us when they are ready to be helped to transition via euthanasia. Animal communication can also be helpful in finding lost pets as the animal does not need to be physically close to the communicator. A recent picture is all a communicator needs to bond with the animal.

I completed all three classes in the beginning of 2010 and I have been on an amazing journey ever since. I had heard of animal communication a few years back but had quickly brushed off the idea, even calling it crazy. I was obviously not ready to receive the gifts and blessings of the Universe, until now.

Ironically, the first pet that became in need of my help after I finished the classes was a cat named Chili Bean, who lived at Lee and Anna's house. Lee called me on a Sunday morning to tell me that Chili suddenly had severe diarrhea. He could not figure out what might have happened since Chili never goes outside and there had been no change in her diet. I offered to communicate with her. Chili communicated to me that she had licked something in the bathroom. She appeared to be a very curious cat. This being my first communication in the real world, I was extremely frightened of being wrong and completely off track. The biggest challenge in learning animal communication is to differentiate what information comes from your imagination as opposed to a true telepathic communication. The imagination is an active process from the brain, whereas communication is a passive process coming from the heart, where you live, feel, see, know and hear with your inner ears the communicated information as if they are real life events truly happening. Since great rewards often come with great risks, I dived in and shared with Chili's family the information I had received. A few hours later, Lee called back ecstatic as he had found the remnant of an aspirin on the bathroom floor. I joined him in celebration! My whole body could finally relax.

When the wife of my co-worker, Jose, became pregnant, Jose brought the very first ultrasound picture for me to communicate with the baby's soul. The energy was truly one of a girl with immense love to give to the world. Not wanting to confirm the sex of the baby until birth, the parents made us wait close to nine months to celebrate my successful communication: Valentina Angelina was the cutest baby girl!

As time passes, I am becoming more confident and more proficient at channeling and interpreting the information. It did not take long for me to start receiving divine and truly powerful messages that were so beautiful that I knew I could not have created them myself. Years of growing will only make us more and more in tune with our inner power and intuition to communicate more and more effectively. Serving the higher good is the ultimate quest, as opposed to trying to feed curiosity. Even though I believe we all have the potential, we certainly do not want everyone to develop it to the same level. It must flow with our life purpose. For some people, learning how to enhance their daily gut feeling and intuition to make sound decisions in face of life's challenges may be all that is required. For others, becoming true mediums and using their skills as a consultant to help other incarnated souls may be required. Often, one's potential may develop further when one reaches a certain age or place in his life. For example, it would have been dangerously overwhelming for me to handle being who I am today during veterinary school. I had enough back then to deal with just basic self-confidence issues. Let's not force anything upon ourselves. Patience is the key. Along the same lines, beware of what you wish for: do you really think you want and can handle hearing the spirits with your physical ears? Or seeing people's aura? How would it benefit you in fulfilling your life mission?

Ever since we moved to Arizona in 2005, Dan and I have wanted to visit Sedona, known as the state's romantic capital. The time finally came soon after finishing the animal communication classes. That is when we learned that Sedona was also known as the Vortex Capital of the world. The timing could not have been better. A vortex in Sedona is a high vibrating place with a spiraling energy flow that facilitates prayer, meditation, communication with the invisible world and healing. We decided to sign up for a vortex tour guided by a Shaman.

My mother and her boyfriend, visiting from Canada, were going to join us at the hotel in Sedona and then continue on their trip afterwards to the Grand Canyon. Dan and I, driving to Sedona from southern Arizona, had decided to camp out in the van like we had done many times before. For us, camping in the van was the ultimate idea of relaxation and ideal vacation: a perfect mix between practicalities and being in touch with nature. We could easily fit a twin size mattress and had several bags hanging from the side walls, all filled with the necessities: clothes, kitchen items and toiletries. We entered the hotel address in our GPS. Due to our late departure, we arrived in Sedona after sunset and following our GPS was mandatory. We arrived at the hotel parking lot (according to the GPS) but failed to see the hotel. We saw some signs – a scenic view, an observatory. By then we realized that our GPS had led us into the parking lot of something beautiful, but what? Our focus had suddenly changed to how peaceful we felt in that place, we felt at home. We did finally find the hotel but decided to go back to the peaceful parking lot we had found to stay for the night. It was not until the next morning that we realized that we were at the bottom of the Bell Rock Vortex. It was breathtaking! We still can not figure out how the GPS made the mistake but what a wonderful mistake it was!

We soon saw the many spiraling trees that live near the vortex and follow its energy flow. I turned on my computer but could barely control the mouse on the screen as it was shaking to the point that I thought something was broken. It is only later that I realized how powerful the vortex vibrations were to interfere with the computer's electromagnetic vibes. My computer was never broken and resumed working normally as soon as we reached a certain distance from the vortex.

During our vortex tour with our Shaman guide, we all felt the powerful energies, stronger or weaker depending of which vortex we were visiting. Everyone's attraction to a particular vortex varied according to one's needs and vibration level. My mother's boyfriend experienced an impressive shamanic energy cleansing session: it was discovered that he had several unresolved past life issues that caused him problems in this current life. As the negative entities were being released from his being, we, including Yogi our dog, felt the urge to move as far away as possible due to the heaviness and negativity of his energies that we could all feel. He reported feeling so much lighter afterwards and feeling more attuned with his soul purpose. Dan and I had the strongest attraction and connection with Bell Rock Vortex. While Dan received a strong visual message from Bell Rock, I was gifted with some powerful words of guidance.

CHAPTER 7

Learning to follow the signs of guidance

I have developed a routine of protection and communion with the Universe with which I always precede a session of animal communication. It begins with looking at the original painting on the cover of this book; I enter into communion with Mother Earth by feeling the roots coming out of my feet entering deep into the Earth to receive guidance but also to give her my love and gratitude. I then raise my arms up to enter into communion with Father Sky and feel the rays of light shining down into my being, making me a divine channel of communication for Universal energy to do its work, to heal our world, for the higher good of the planet and its habitants, including all of nature's creations and creatures. In doing this, I surrender all control and truly become an instrument to receive messages from the animals, the spirit world and the Universe, for healing of all beings. I then enter into communication with the living creature in need of help, by bonding with its energy via a recent picture. I welcome his messages of guidance, but I also welcome any beneficial information provided by his subconscious mind, about past lives for example, or messages from his Angels and soul family members, for the greater good.

I believe that the information that comes across is always filtered by higher powers. We are all unique beings, and therefore, we are all unique channels of communication. I can recall vividly two communications where the animals shared selected information with me but were reluctant to share certain other information, showing me clearly where my place was in helping their families. Some answers were not for me to know or else the timing was not right for the family to access this information.

It was hard at first to let go of the need to give everyone a happy ending and fix everyone's problems. I have come to the realization that pain and obstacles are necessary for the growth of the soul. Illnesses and life challenges are wake up calls with the purpose of bringing motivation and action in improving something in one's life. We must accept that the information that comes through at a particular time is what is needed for growth. If I can not give someone an answer about something, there is a reason that is, whether we figure it out now or only later.

Along the same lines, everything in our lives happens for a reason and teaches us a lesson. As an example, I will compare two families each with a sick puppy that is battling the life-threatening disease of parvovirus. In the first case, the family has limited income and genuinely cares for the puppy who they just rescued from a bad situation. This puppy makes a rapid recovery without the need to be hospitalized, saving the family a lot of worry and money.

The other family decides to skip the puppy's vaccinations and instead buys a large, expensive flat screen television. I think in this instance the Universe is trying to teach this family a very important lesson, which is that caring for the puppy is more important than owning a "thing". I can see how this puppy may require several days of hospitalization costing a lot of money in medical care. The puppy might even die in spite of all the best efforts of the medical team, if this is the only way that the family will learn the lesson. It only takes a slight shift in energy, in the family's emotions, to provoke the shift in the puppy's body, either positive or negative. Again, everything happens for a reason. Everyone we meet, animal or human, has a lesson for us and offers us an opportunity to grow into becoming a better being.

This shows that you can try your best to help someone and do things right but you ultimately do not have complete control over the outcome of their situation. Again, depending on what deeper lessons there are to be learned (I call it the "jinx" factor that we all bring upon ourselves at times), things will go wrong in spite of someone's best effort to help. Illustrating this point, I will tell you the story of Benny: Benny was a very old and sweet dog. I went to his home to assist him in transitioning peacefully. He fell asleep smoothly with the first injection of sedative. However, when I gave him the euthanasia solution, he remained asleep without leaving his body. I had to give him three doses for him to finally pass. Mom confessed that the same thing had happened to her feline friend a few years back and that she was blaming herself for both instances. Mom had a huge need to control and needed everything to be perfect. She realized that night that she had to let go as we often can not control things in our lives. In this scenario, I was only the instrument through which she would learn such a valuable lesson.

In my experience, life becomes much easier once you surrender this need for control and learn to listen to and follow the Universe's guidance through signs sent to us – the so-called coincidences and messages of synchronicity that most people brush off so quickly in their daily lives. This concept has clearly been described in *The Celestine Prophecy* written by James Redfield. This book explains how the Universe sends us signs and messages of guidance to help us make decisions, change or improve something in our life and get back on the right path of fulfilling our incarnation. While some can come to us in dreams, a lot of these messages are given to us by other unwitting people.

Another example of this synchronicity was the time when I arrived at Sun Bear's home. Mom immediately noticed the dragonfly trinket sticking out of my pants pocket. It had accidentally gotten hooked as opposed to dropping inside my pocket with the rest of my key chain. This dragonfly spoke strongly to mom and brought her peace that she was making the right decision in helping her best friend transition. It also brought her relief that I was the right person to help them. When I walked in the house, I noticed several dragonfly picture hangings. Mom also shared that she had a large dragonfly tattooed on her back as it was her animal totem.

I also find Koko's story fascinating: Koko was a thirteen-year-old Sharpei mix. She had an abdominal tumor and a large skin mass. Although Koko had slowed down somewhat, she was still interested in eating and her quality of life was judged adequate. On the Fourth of July holiday, her watermelon-size skin mass started bleeding. Mom and her husband, who believed it was time to help her transition, called me. When I arrived at their home, Koko's mass was no longer bleeding and mom was very upset for getting so alarmed. Mom felt extremely torn between helping Koko transition now, or waiting for another time. I could tell that Koko was uncomfortable. Her gums were pale and her abdomen was significantly enlarged and rock hard. Additionally, her skin mass was very big and impaired Koko's ability to lie on her side. Although the mass had stopped bleeding temporarily, it most likely would bleed again, due to the fact that her skin had become extremely fragile from the stretching of the tumor. During our conversation, mom revealed that they had adopted Koko thirteen years before, during the Fourth of July holiday weekend. I became speechless to the huge coincidence this was. Weighing all our options, mom and I decided to help her transition now, as we knew that Koko was going to continue to decline and was not going to let go on her own. Immediately after her passing, her skin mass resumed bleeding, and released a large amount of fluid. Speechless to this second strong sign sent into their lives, I was so happy for Koko's family to receive the confirmation to have made the right decision for their beloved friend.

Guided by their pictures, I have received messages from the Universe and Angels for my mother, my brother, my eight-month-old godson as well as for a few of my friends and co-workers. Every time, my loved one connects strongly with the message destined to guide him or her onto the path of self-realization and fulfillment.

Here are a few important lessons that I have learned from animals through communication:

1. Respect for the deceased animals and the spirit world

During our animal communication classes, we performed the exercise of communicating with a deceased animal we knew. However, I learned quickly from Hayley's spirit not to bother the spirit world unless there is real trouble and genuine help is needed. Hayley appeared extremely busy in guiding my husband from up above and her message to me was clear: stay back. I also received a similar message from Moses' spirit as he seemed busy preparing to reincarnate into a small dog. He did, however, advise us to offer Nuru the option of wearing his old collar to gain strength and confidence. Four years after Moses' transition, Nuru is still struggling, feeling like a "fragile flower lost at sea." We are trying our best to give her the guidance and support that she needs in order to define her own identity.

Since these two experiences, I am very cautious in reaching out to deceased animals and understand the disrespect of trying to receive information out of curiosity. It must serve a higher purpose, a healing purpose. The only time I now attempt to communicate with deceased animals is when there is a real need down here, to help the grieving family heal and get closure. In those instances, the energy is very different as I feel welcomed and receive beautiful messages, which I did from three canine companions: Rowdy wanted mom to know that he will be coming back into her life in a new physical body; TeJana told her dad that she was his spiritual mother and asked him to keep her living through him; and Charlie, who had such a strong husband energy, instructed mom that he was going to remain by her side and help her accomplish her projects.

2. Some pets were humans in their previous incarnation

Some pets that I have communicated with have a very strong human energy. I recall Becky Lou's energy of a grandmother whereas Kona was a lonely man who suffered greatly from betrayal in his previous life. Tata feels like a human in a dog's body, said that her name was Veronica and that she has walked the Earth with her family before.

I have read in the book *Animal Voices, Telepathic Communication in the Web of Life*, by Dawn Baumann Brunke, that humans can indeed reincarnate into animals' bodies and vice versa. Depending of one's incarnation purpose, a human can decide to come back, for example, as a guinea pig, to go through the process of giving birth quicker than in a human body, if this is the area targeted for soul growth. I have quite a few clients who also feel that their dogs were humans before, so much so these pets relate more to other people than other dogs. I will always remember the story of one of my clients, whose Poodle preferred to sit on the bench at the dog park with the dog owners and watch the other dogs play, rather than play with the dogs.

Bella is a young Schnauzer with a huge personality. Mom adopted her a few years after the passing of her husband. She quickly noticed how Bella would selectively bite certain people she met. Mom was stunned to realize that she was in fact biting the people that her husband had always disliked or had distrusted. When I started my communication with Bella, I could not believe how strong and masculine her energy was. There was no doubt in my mind that she was the owner's deceased husband. I learned that he had reincarnated to learn tolerance of others. Mom confirmed that her husband had deep trust issues, therefore, my communication made sense to her. Mom also sent me a picture of her husband which I only had to take a rapid look at to feel the same intense and distrusting energy – it was Bella's soul.

The owner of my canine patient Goofey is a medium and believes strongly that Goofey's soul has visited her before in the previous dog she had, also named Goofey. The current Goofey would in fact only respond to her previous name. That is why mom decided to keep her same name during this second incarnation. Magic's mom, also an intuitive, knew that her bird would come back as a cat. When she recognized him in a feral cat racing by her house, she called him by his soul name and Magic came to a complete stop. They reunited and lived a wonderful life together. I have encountered five or six other families with similar stories: one's cat was her horse, one's dog was his donkey, and one client was convinced that her cat was her reincarnated grandfather. Furthermore, one client believes that her pet's soul will return to Earth within six months, while a dog communicated to me that he would return as a horse to continue with mom where they had left off.

Many people experience a powerful attraction to a specific person, of the same or opposite sex, or a powerful attraction to a specific animal without understanding the reason for such an attraction. I believe that we are attracted to the soul living inside the physical body, whatever the physical body looks like at the time. Again, we often reincarnate with the same souls. Our change in physical bodies can make it rather challenging to recognize each other, which is why we must follow our feelings.

3. Knowing your pet's life mission helps you grow

A life mission is not the same for all pets, and one must be aware that it can be anything. Abby's life mission is to open daddy's heart and teach him that the most important in life is spending time with your loved ones; because of this, she constantly becomes sick to get his attention. Java, an over-the-top happy and difficult to train chocolate

Labrador, teaches her family that everything is possible when we put our mind to it; dear Pia, with her unique personality, teaches her family unconditional love; Thorn's teachings are to always look at the bright side of life, to be happy and to enjoy life and your loved ones as opposed to waste time being upset at one another. Swayze is the incarnation of patience and teaches everyone on his path tolerance, love and harmony and that everybody makes mistakes. What matters is that people are trying their best. He advises us not to get angry when someone makes a mistake, but to be patient while they learn and grow, and always send them your love.

4. Animals have emotions

Several pets have told me how much they hate to hear us argue because it frightens and stresses them. Kabo is a horse extremely sensitive to loud voices and anger. He finds it soothing to have loving words whispered into his ears. Several pets have also shared how they dislike when people force them into being picked up or rubbed on their bodies in unwanted places. They like things to be done on their own terms. They like to be asked first for permission, as a sign of respect, before we do anything to them. Ask your pets out loud before you pick them up. Watch their body language for the answer, or feel it in your heart. Animals are asking us to do to them what they enjoy, for their pleasure, not for ours. Be patient and go slow with your pets. Learn from them.

Additionally, animals feel the energy when we make belittling and/or negative comments about them or laugh at them in front of our friends. They can become really upset, and lose confidence and self-esteem.

5. Know the personalities of the animals in your life to understand them better

It can be extremely insightful to get details about each pet in your household. The feline Lucy has the "Mom" attitude. She is the supervisor of the group, needing to know all that is happening at all times, taking care of everyone and making sure that everyone is alright, people and animals. When Jake and Caesar transitioned, it brought her peace to be told that they were in a better place and felt healthy again. She was finally able to stop worrying about them. She calls the other cats at home "the kids". Her message to them was: "Behave, I'm watching you". One of her housemates, Dusty, thinks that everything in life is a game. He does not like rules and thinks Lucy is too serious. During my communication with him I had trouble keeping him focused because he only wanted to play. Although I was able to convince the felines Yuki and Celine to stop chewing electrical cords in the house, in exchange of increased attention and play times for Celine, and by providing Yuki with a type of treats that he used to love playing with and eating, Dusty did not agree to compromise. His family will need to be firm at reprimanding him when he chews, otherwise he will think they are playing a game.

Some animals appear to be "young souls" as they seem to never mature and want to play their whole lives, like Dusty and Chili Bean. There are also animals that are "old souls", the wise ones that seem to have an incredible amount of wisdom like Boullie and Shirley. Some pets are also extremely empathic and always bring support to the animal or human in distress like Poseidon. Our own feline friend Sunny is our most empathic pet. When his older sister Munchie became acutely blind, he immediately sat next to her to bring her comfort. In fact, Munchie would watch the sunset every night. That night that she became blind, Sunny kept her company for the first time and they "watched" the sunset together.

6. Many pets' behavioral problems are caused by us

The feline Marguerite started defecating on her dad's pillow to remind him that she exists and needs his company. This was her way to get his attention and tell him that she misses him. The feline Tammy was hoping for the same response when he started urinating on dad's side of the bed. However, most people do not spend time trying to understand the meaning of such behaviors. Unfortunately, most people become angry, resent their pets and relinquish them to shelters. For these pets, this becomes a second rejection causing deep emotional wounds. Can you imagine how these animals feel, when all they wanted was to give and receive love? Behavioral problems are the number one reason that animals are abandoned in shelters.

The animals with behavioral issues are the ones who need our help the most. Again, most behavioral problems are caused by us in the first place because we are not providing our pets with appropriate stimulation and attention, leading them to boredom, lack of fulfillment and development of undesirable behaviors. Furthermore, just like many pets will grieve the loss of a companion, relinquishing a pet to the shelter and separating him from a best friend can have severe health repercussions for either separated pets, as it was the case for Louise and Papa.

I helped a dog named Red that was panting constantly secondary to emotional distress. He had trouble keeping up with mom's unstable lifestyle. He described it as a circus with no routine or down times: "Life is going too fast, like a race, and I am out of breath trying to keep up". Thoughts were racing in his mind. Red was completely mirroring his owner. Mom confessed that the information was exact and started bringing routine and organization into her life, therefore restoring sanity for her companion and herself.

More pets have shared this need for calm, peace, stability and routine. It appears that the fast pace of life caused by our modern society bothers our pets, understandably. Following a routine helps them know what is going to happen next, which decreases their anxiety. Disorder and lack of cleanliness also bother some pets, who will urinate inappropriately in a cluttered environment secondary to feeling lost and disorganized. Marking the territory is an attempt for them to regain that lost territory.

I have come across wonderful books called *Whale Done! The Power of Positive Relationships* and *Whale Done! Parenting*. Both are written by Kenneth Blanchard, Ph.D and his team of whale trainers at SeaWorld. These books have confirmed my theories that animals are just like humans and vice versa. The books are intended to teach people how to raise their human children as well as how to develop positive relationships with other people in their lives, based on the animal model. I can only hope that everyone reads them to deepen their understanding of the same emotional nature of humans and animals: we all respond to the same stimuli; we are all looking for pleasure; a person or animal learns much faster when the process is fun; a person or animal loves praises and rewards and will repeat the behavior that led to them; the teacher must set the student up for success by giving him all the tools he needs to perform the asked behavior or task; redirect a negative behavior to the correct behavior and focus on that positive behavior (positive reinforcement). The books also suggest finding and enhancing natural abilities and passions in everyone, animal or human. For example, not all horses love to race, not all dogs want to play frisbee, nor do all children want to become doctors or lawyers. The earlier we detect what someone is passionate about, the easier it is to support him in developing and enhancing his skills further, leading to ultimate satisfaction and happiness. Who wants to be forced into doing something they hate? Empathic animals, just like empathic people, are the happiest working in close contact with other living souls, like therapists. Whereas athletic horses that love to compete will be ecstatic training hard and racing on a regular basis, just like professional hockey players and Olympic athletes. It is extremely destructive for both animals and people to be forced into doing something when motivation and pleasure are absent. Performing out of love and fun is much healthier than performing out of fear. Recognize, support and respect everyone's passion, like you want others to recognize, support and respect yours.

CHAPTER 8

Fascinating communications

1. Rolli

My cousin called me in tears when her sweet cat, Rolli, escaped from her house and got lost outside. Although it had already been several days, I believed that he was not too far, close to a pink brick walled house. My cousin posted flyers everywhere and did find a couple of houses similar to the one I had described in her neighborhood. As I was preparing to leave my house a few days later when Rolli had been missing for over a week, I developed a knot in my stomach, a feeling telling me that Rolli had found a new home and that his life mission involved staying with his new family. I was desperately trying to convince myself that this could not be, however, I knew that I had to call my cousin promptly. I began crying as I was telling her that she had to let him go. I cried even more when I heard my cousin cry. From my communication, Rolli seemed happy, and therefore my cousin reluctantly accepted letting him live his life. Children, humans or animals, are not ours to keep. They each have their life mission to fulfill as well. Although guidance and safety is important, parents must ultimately allow their loved ones to be free and fulfill their own life mission.

The very next day, my cousin received a phone call from a neighbor who had found Rolli. She raced over to him and brought him back home. My initial reaction was to feel defeated in my skills of communicator. However, I quickly started wondering if the chain of events would have been different if my cousin had not learned the valuable lesson of surrendering control and respecting everyone's life purpose. The timing was certainly impeccable: as soon as my cousin's energies shifted to letting go, Rolli reappeared. We may never know for sure but most importantly, Rolli has returned home and my cousin has grown into a better person through this experience.

2. Grandpa's visit

A few months ago, I had a communication with my deceased grandfather that started as a dream: I was frightened by a large insect that was attached to my chest and he was guiding me in how to remove it safely. As I began to wake up, I remember asking him if there was anything we could do for my grandmother. Since his transition a couple of years ago, she had felt very lonely and the children have had mixed feelings about how to care for her. He told me that all she needed from everyone was always to be loved. He also asked me to tell her that he loved her very much. As he held me in his arms and gave me the most wonderful hug, I woke up fully.

I felt confused as I tried to understand what had happened. Was it all a dream? It felt so real at the end like he had really visited from the spirit world. Why would he come visit me all of a sudden? I immediately called my mother in Canada to make sure everything was well. Right away she proceeded to tell me that they were almost done moving my grandmother into an assisted-living home. Tears of heavenly joy and gratitude were running down my cheeks as I was telling my mother that grandpa had really visited me and that he was obviously moving in with grandma. He wanted to make sure she knew how much he loved her and that he was still by her side.

3. Blake & Jake

Blake and Jake, indoor cats and brothers, had been urinating inappropriately around the house for several weeks. I learned through my communication that Blake was a leader, a loner, a very dominant and independent cat. His biggest problem was his frustration to being locked inside and among so many other cats. Urinating was his way of trying to claim his territory. More importantly however, he deeply wanted to live outside. Life was happening and he was not a part of it. He was watching it go by through the window.

On the other hand, his brother Jake was the follower and would urinate wherever Blake did. Jake had self-confidence issues and a constant need for guidance from other pets and people. Jake was too fearful to be outdoors. He was satisfied inside, as long as he had a leader to follow.

Three months went by and life had become really good for everyone: Blake was allowed outside and would actually come in and out as he pleased, Jake had found a new leader in the household, the inappropriate urination subsided, so the family was happy. After a few days of Blake not reporting to the house, mom became worried and asked me to communicate with him again. Blake shared that he had left his physical body and was happier than ever. Although mom and I felt bad, Blake taught us an important lesson: the goal of life is to be happy. Blake was happy outside. He was so grateful that we allowed him to live the life that he wanted to live, which is the ultimate gift to someone. Blake had a shorter life but a good one as he said. He was free and happy. He was eaten by wildlife and felt at peace with the outcome. Being a cat was not easy. He was happy to have participated in the circle of life by giving the coyote a good meal. We all come to this Earth alone and leave alone. One must take risks to gain happiness sometimes.

Again, everyone has a life mission and a purpose for being here. Animals do, too. We must be fair to other living creatures and listen to their needs. There is a fine line between safety and boredom. I do believe that most reptiles, spiders, fish and turtles kept in aquariums would be much happier and fulfilled living in the outside world where stimulation and entertainment are constant. This is true for several birds, hamsters, rabbits, guinea pigs, as well as cats. The widely accepted syndrome of the indoor-declawed-fat-bored cat is the not the answer to our problem as I believe several of these cats are "existing" as opposed to "living". Of course life is safer if you never leave your house, but it can be extremely boring and unfulfilling. One must be allowed to follow one's destiny. Stagnation and lack of fulfillment lead to stress and disease. How would you like to be caged when you can run, fly and swim in the wild? I am living proof of this concept: a child must fly from the nest, sometimes far away, to find fulfillment and happiness. Sometimes you fall, you get hurt, but you get back up, stronger, wiser and continue your journey squeezing every drop of happiness out of life. Doing so, you are not only existing, but you are truly living your life to the fullest. I am grateful that my parents understood my needs and prefer to see me happy far away from them, rather than safe and unfulfilled close to them.

4. Muse & Dude

Muse and Little Dude were two feline brothers living together. Muse had begun marking around the house with his urine several months before. I first met Muse when he came into the hospital to be euthanized. Reviewing his records, I learned that he was given several courses of different anti-anxiety medications without success. After months of trials and frustration, Muse's family decided that they could not accept his marking behavior anymore. Having just finished the animal communication classes, I really wanted to try helping this family. Was I too late? I could not believe that I might not have a chance to save Muse from being euthanized. This was a touchy situation as the family had already made up their mind about letting Muse go. When I entered the examination room, I saw that dad had come alone and that because he loved Muse so much, it was difficult to say goodbye to him. I felt so torn inside, my heart was pounding in my chest. Do I say something? Or do I regret it forever? I finally took a huge risk and offered to communicate with Muse to see what the problem was. To my huge relief, dad accepted.

By communicating with Muse, I learned that his marking was due to issues with his feline brother. Muse felt loved by both mom and dad but felt very oppressed by his brother. By marking, he was trying to claim his territory, taking his place and showing that he exists. My conversation with Dude confirmed it. However, the first thing that Dude told me was that he deeply disliked to be called Little Dude (which was his official name). He much preferred being called Dude and so we all acquiesced to his wishes. Dude then told me how much he resented Muse and was jealous of him. He saw Muse as the favorite child, therefore, would bully him out of frustration, wishing he could make him disappear and become the number one cat.

Mom and dad were completely speechless about the accuracy of the information received. They confessed favoring Muse over Dude and agreed to give Dude more attention as requested. Everyone understood each other's feelings and forgave each other, agreeing to make changes so everyone could become happier. The situation greatly improved for about six months.

However, when things worsened again, Dude communicated that he was still jealous of Muse, wishing he were him, the center of attention and the number one cat. The only way that he was going to be happy would be by not seeing Muse at all. He would even be happier moving into a new home, ideally with a man. Muse still felt oppressed and was unable to shine and be himself. During the time we tried hard to find Dude a new home, Muse became sick and succumbed to an acute illness a couple of months later. While mom and dad were saddened by his loss, Dude finally became number one and is now happier than ever.

5. Molly

Molly is a wonderful nine-year-old Golden-Labrador mix who lives in Canada with my sister. Molly was rescued as a puppy and extremely well trained by the age of one year. She was mom's best friend and became the flower girl at our wedding. Unfortunately, after my sister got married herself, having children became the priority and time spent with Molly became scarce. Nevertheless, every night Molly would sleep at the foot of the master bed. Over one year ago, suddenly, Molly was found sleeping alone in the living room. Mom was considering giving her up, realizing how little time she had for Molly anymore. When I communicated with Molly, I asked her if she would like to go live with one of her mom's friend that Molly knew. She became so terribly sad to the idea that I started crying profusely. Molly explained how devastated she would feel not having her routine, her home and her feline friends anymore. Molly had pretty much raised a cat named Charlotte and she would be heartbroken not seeing her everyday. Molly understood that her mom's priorities had changed since the children came along. I did explain to Molly that she was still loved very much and had her place at the foot of the bed. The next day, my sister called to tell me that Molly had slept at the foot of the bed. It has now been over a year and she is still sleeping at the foot of the bed every night.

6. Kona

Kona is a four-year-old German shepherd. His mom is very sweet natured and has raised multiple dogs of the same breed over the years. Mom adopted Kona as a puppy and quickly realized that he had severe aggression issues towards people and animals. While mom talked to veterinarians and several trainers, no one could help. What I learned from Kona was truly fascinating. It appeared that his fear of strangers (people and animals) came from the fact that he had been let down in the past. He had been taken advantage of, as well as hurt and betrayed. Trusting others was a big deal. All of this comes from a past life when he was a human.

As a human, he had chosen to end his life due to the difficulties he was facing: abandonment, lack of love and self-worth. By returning in a dog's body, this could not happen again, therefore, he would have to persevere through the difficulties. This is also his message to the world: we all can make the change, the mental and emotional shift, to work in the positive, as opposed to letting ourselves go to negative places: drugs, addictions, theft, homicide. We decide which path we take, the positive one or the negative one. It starts with loving ourselves and fighting for our happiness. Don't be a victim, be a leader. Kona is the symbol of hope, his color is green.

For the first time, I was given a healing color for an animal. I instructed mom to visualize him in the middle of a beautiful shining green cloud. The people whose lives he will touch the most are, indeed, the homeless, the prisoners and people with fragile minds like his that need a ray of hope and an example of perseverance, courage, self-love and self-esteem. Kona, once healed, can then start teaching the world and be the strong and powerful leader that he is.

7. Sissy

Sissy was a very ill cat rescued from the shelter. Right away, mom asked me to communicate with her: Sissy comes from "the heart of the Universe". She irradiates love. Love is stronger than anything. She is here to help heal our world with love. Immediately, the song "All You Need is Love", by the Beatles started playing in my head. I knew this song would be a very powerful tool for mom to heal from what was happening to Sissy.

Sissy teaches us to stay in the positive. When I asked questions like why she got sick or about her past, she would always bring me back to NOW and LOVE. All she needs is love. I told her that we would like to try giving her antibiotics and fluids in the hope that she would feel better and she accepted. I was not able to get an answer to how long she was going to stay with us but she said that it did not matter. What was important was our feelings and to heal our world with love. No matter what, give love to everyone. The people that cause the most hurt are the ones who need the most love.

Interestingly, I had found a rock in my yard a few days before Sissy came into my life and I had called it the "heart of the Universe". It was pink and shaped like a heart. I felt strongly about holding the rock in my hand when I communicated with Sissy. I quickly realized that this rock was a part of her as it represented what she was here to teach. I also felt strongly that the rock needed to be reunited with Sissy and mom, so I brought it to them. I also received a message from the Universe for mom, which was that her soul purpose was also to give LOVE, which was all that the Universe needed her to do.

Another fascinating coincidence is that mom had lost a dear feline friend, Ms. Tess, from heart disease, several months before rescuing Sissy. Her passing was unexpected and mom felt guilty to not have been at her side. Several months later, her powerful attraction for Sissy was unexplained but she knew she had to take her home. Amazingly enough, Sissy allowed Merry to relive Ms. Tess' transition by having heart disease herself. This time, mom was able to be by Sissy's side when she transitioned, allowing her to finally find closure and peace. Thank you Sissy!

CHAPTER 9

Why do we get sick?

My life experiences have taught me that this is a question with several answers. Although these answers can sometimes be challenging to sort through, it is possible:

1. DIET: You and your pet are what you eat. Someone who eats fast foods, processed and preservative-filled foods is at a higher health risk compared to someone who eats high quality, free range meat, fresh fruits and vegetables, or else who has a complete vegan diet. For our pets, there is a wide variety of diets available. While some are wonderful, some are truly comparable to the fast foods that people eat. Again, food should look as much as possible like how nature gives it to us: an apple should look like an apple: raw, organic, not processed.

I had the pleasure of reading *Le premier des Hurons* (The first of the Hurons), a book written by the French Canadian Grand Chef Max Gros-Louis. I was delighted to learn that mosquitoes and other parasites were more attracted to his people when they were eating the cheap and preservative-filled cans of food brought by the Palefaces, as opposed to when they were eating their traditional and natural diet consisting of wild fresh meat and fresh corn. My life experiences also support this theory, as I have found that a higher quality diet helps prevent flea and tick infestations on dogs and cats.

2. LIFESTYLE: Smoking, sleep deprivation, lack of physical exercise, overexposure to electromagnetic vibes like computers, cell phones and television, can all lead to illness.

3. ENVIRONMENT: Some people and animals are very impacted by their environment: noise pollution, allergies, city life versus country life, contagious diseases, sun-induced skin and eye diseases like cancer, lupus and keratitis in both humans and animals.

4. GENETIC: We all look like our parents. There are several undesirable genes that lead to inherited physical and mental illnesses among humans and animals. Unfortunately, when it comes to animals, we have created and worsened a lot of these diseases by breeding for looks as opposed to breeding for health. If we would watch how Mother Nature does wonders using natural selection, we would realize that it is truly the path to follow. From one generation to the next, the individuals better adapted to their environment survive better, reproduce better and therefore pass their superior genes to the next generation, while the less desirable and weaker genes disappear.

Flat noses, floppy ears and bulging eyes may be cute features; however, they do lead to more physical problems. With hip dysplasia, impaired breathing and insufficient temperature regulation, skin allergies and whelping difficulties, the English bulldog is far from being as healthy as the spunky coyote with his long nose, straight ears and strong bones. With his excessive amount of fur leading to life-threatening hair ball problems, flat nose, chronic eye and nasal problems, dental disease and challenge in grasping food, the man made Persian feline is also far from being as well adapted and healthy as its wild cousins. Let's be fair to animals by breeding for their health!

5. STRESS AND EMOTIONS: Here are a few simple examples of how the mind is in close relationship with the physical body: sadness leads to tears; happiness leads to laughter; a week of final exams often leads to stomach ache and gastrointestinal upset; stress prior to a visit to the dentist or public speaking may lead to increased heart rate and immense sweats; hearing the news that a loved one was in an car accident turns your stomach into a knot and your skin blemishes. A friend of mine lost his house and became hypertensive, which no medication could control. Another close friend, Melanie, developed diabetes secondary to her parents divorcing.

Birds are extremely sensitive to stress and can die quickly just from being examined. The same is true for feral cats. I have witnessed how performing a nail trim on an eighteen-year-old frail feline can lead to its collapse. Among the several dogs boarding at a kennel while their owners are away, those that perceive it as a great place of fun will have a wonderful time. However, the ones feeling stressed, abandoned and worried about the separation from their families will be the ones developing stress colitis and diarrhea. Addison's disease is a well recognized condition in people and dogs described as an insufficient production of stress hormones by the body. Those affected individuals are therefore extremely sensitive to stress, which can cause life-threatening collapse and even death when the disease is not well controlled.

Boredom, lack of stimulation and lack of fulfillment are also common causes of illness among people and animals. Cats need much more stimulation than we think. Boredom in dogs leads to behavioral problems like barking, chewing inappropriate objects and digging holes. Boredom often also leads to aggression when cats can not fulfill their instinctive need to hunt, or else pets may "eat their emotions" like people do and become very overweight. Again, there is a fine line between feeling safe and being bored. Each animal has a unique personality and unique needs. For example, Marilyn was found living near a friend's house as a feral cat. After years of feeding her, she finally entered the house and now sleeps in bed with her new family. The house door can remain wide open but Marilyn enjoys her new life too much to ever wanting to step outside again.

The key is to find an adequate balance between safety and happiness for each of our pets. This includes lots of play time and mental stimulation for our furry friends. Playing hide and seek (cats love it too!), or spending supervised time outside in an enclosed area can be ways to achieve such a balance. One of the toys that our cats enjoy immensely is a guitar string. When I am pressed for time to play, I tie a long string to my waist or else hold it in my hand as I perform the chores around the house. It never takes long for my feline friends to start chasing me around. The best cat toy is obviously a live mammal to hunt, like a mouse. Unfortunately, domestication has led our tamed feline friends to hunt on a full stomach, therefore for pleasure, as opposed to hunting for survival like they would if living in the wild. Hunting for pleasure causes much greater suffering to the prey animals.

Any negative emotions like fear, oppression, anger, resentment, guilt and regret will eventually lead to illness if left unprocessed and bottled up. It is normal to experience these emotions. However, we must process them quickly, express them and release them to allow our vital energy to flow again. Anytime I feel heavy or I feel a "knot" in my stomach, I must take a step back, figure out where the feeling is coming from and take the appropriate steps to release it, restoring inner peace, harmony and the feeling of lightness. We may not be able to prevent feeling negative emotions from time to time but we can all decide how we react to them. Blaming others and playing the victim only leads to more emotional hurt and makes us waste precious time and energy. Choose to feel as good as you can in the face of any situation in life and stay in the positive. Find ways to release any negative emotion. Change your perception of a situation, and remember that no one can hurt us with their words but that we choose to let those words hurt us. Talk to the person who caused you to be upset, cry if you need to and scream if you need to. Negative feelings that are not expressed outwardly will become expressed inwardly, in the physical body.

On the other hand, positive emotions like having the pleasure of watching animals cuddle together can lead to relaxation of the whole body and decrease in blood pressure. Learning to take situations with a grain of salt is very healing. One must learn to laugh at oneself. Too many people take life too seriously and get self-conscious when they realize that they did something really silly. See life as a game and learn to play it. When you make a silly mistake, give yourself a break, laugh at yourself and grow from it. Laughter is by far the best medicine.

6. CHINESE MEDICINE: Practitioners link illness to six different causes: environment, season, diet, lack of exercise, imbalanced lifestyle and emotions.

7. PAST LIFE: This involves unresolved issues, like we have discussed before, and that can lead to problems in our current life. Interestingly, the medium Sylvia Browne explains in her book, *Blessings From the Other Side,* how birth marks on people represent an area of trauma in a previous life.

8. FEEDING OFF SOMEONE ELSE/MIRRORING SOMEONE:
I have quickly realized during my career that when someone has multiple pets, the first one to get sick and pass away is often the one that the owner loved the most, hence the one who spent the most time with the owner, absorbing his energies. I have also noticed how some animals age much faster than others. For example, a sixteen-year-old Chihuahua may still be in perfect health while a ten-year-old of the same breed is dying of chronic renal failure and his coat has turned completely gray. I strongly believe that taking negative emotional baggage from their owner leads to accelerated aging and deterioration of the pet's physical body. Interestingly, I have seen multiple situations where the owner and his pet share the same diseases: bladder stones, back problems, cancer, inflammatory bowel disease and more. One of my clients, Karina, made the realization that everyone at home had chronic foot problems of all kinds: her son, her dog and herself. In two dogs, Bella and Yogi, I have seen how their extremely anxious owners triggered the apparition of a benign growth on their skin called a histiocytoma.

9. GETTING YOUR ENERGY DRAINED OR POLLUTED BY SOMEONE ELSE: Interacting with some people leaves you feeling very drained. Everyone has experienced it. A child may develop chronic ear infections when subconsciously trying to block off the noise pollution of his parents' constant arguing that he no longer wants to hear. It is vital to remove the people that are depleting your energy, bringing you down and "polluting you" from your life.

10. NOT BEING IN TUNE WITH YOUR LIFE MISSION: If you are not on your path of fulfilling your life mission, you will eventually receive a wake up call, and hopefully, you will recognize it. An illness or trauma can be a sign that you are doing something wrong and a change is needed in your life to restore your vital flow of energy. A friend of mine, Glen, suffered from a stroke as he was reaching into his pocket for his wallet to buy cigarettes. For him, the timing could not have been more perfect and the message clearer: it is time to stop procrastinating, to stop smoking and to care for your body.

An illness can also be a way to lead you to meeting a key person that will impact your life and help you find your career or realize your dreams and passions, therefore being in tune with your life mission. I will always remember how the feline Sycamore, through his natural death following a long-lasting illness, taught his owner Shelby, a ten-year-old child, to become a veterinarian. In another example, Sushi, a feline with severe behavioral problems, led mom and me to discussing animal communication, which then sparked the interest of Sushi's favorite family member, a young girl who was already showing aptitudes for energy healing.

I developed a low grade tonsillitis that lasted several months a few years ago. The timing of its healing coincided perfectly with me singing at my sister's wedding. The throat represents self-expression, therefore, diseases to the throat are often linked to lack of self-expression. In my case, singing was a childhood dream that I had pushed aside. Subconsciously, it appeared to have caused me sadness. Singing at my sister's wedding allowed me to fulfill this dream and my throat healed.

11. PART OF SOUL CONTRACT: You may have agreed in your life contract to receive an illness in order to teach and impact others' lives around you. Examples of this may include cases where babies and children become ill. Additionally, these young souls may have agreed to an early return to the spirit world as soon as their mission was accomplished. When our cat Munchie became acutely blind, my communication revealed that its purpose was to teach her family unity. Reflecting on the time when it happened, we could only agree that her blindness had led Dan and me into shifting our energies and working as a team that was stronger than ever. It also reminded us to appreciate what we have and focus only on what is truly important in life: our loved ones.

12. UNCATEGORIZED: Other situations are difficult to categorize, however, they are worthy of mention. People can become sick when subconsciously wishing to avoid performing a certain disliked task. Getting sick gives them a reason for not fulfilling an obligation. Along the same lines, someone who feels guilty for taking time off will develop an illness to feel "allowed" to relax and rest. People who are working too much and do not know when to stop will also bring upon themselves an illness to teach them that work is not everything in life. People (especially children) and animals, like one of my patients Abby, may constantly get sick to gain more attention from their family.

My mother, Ginette, has helped a client understand why one of her twin boys was constantly sick from a young age. Sorting out her emotions, the lady remembered how during her pregnancy she became extremely overwhelmed when she learned that she was carrying twins. She was scared of not being able to care for two babies. One of the boys perceived it as rejection from his mother, therefore, was subconsciously trying to disappear ever since he was born. Once these emotions became known, the sick boy was finally able to start healing.

Professional help from mediums, intuitives, life coaches, shamans, hypnotists, therapists and doctors may be needed to sort out the cause of your illness. But more often than not, the best person to figure out why an illness, trauma or life situation happens and what it is here to teach you, is yourself. In all situations, an illness is intended for growth of the soul, and therefore, is beneficial.

The Universe wants to make sure that we notice the message it is sending us. Life has taught me that most people tend to injure their writing hand, driving foot or guitar-playing hand. In my experience, we initially receive small signs, however, those quickly grow if the person targeted is not learning the lesson fast enough. Someone who fails to learn from a small incident is asking for a bigger life challenge to happen. Remember that a small injury may be a huge blessing in disguise if it prevents you from greater suffering as things can always get worse. Unfortunately, the more time that lapses, the harder it becomes to sort through years and years of ignored life lessons. Additionally, the physical body may reach a point of extreme overload where the mind can no longer process the teachings. Death may occur at this point, assuring the soul a next incarnation to work on the same life lessons, which hopefully can be learned faster.

"Total Biology of Living Beings" is a concept developed in Europe by two medical doctors, Dr. Ryke Geerd Hamer and Dr. Claude Sabbah. It originated in 1978. Its main premise is the scientifically proven relationship between the psyche, the brain and the body. It teaches us to become aware of the emotional trauma behind any physical condition. The type of emotional response, therefore how humans and animals react to situations in life, decides what disease becomes created and where it occurs in the physical body. For example, the loss of a job: the person who perceives it as a huge loss will develop a mass; the one who overflows with anger will develop ulcers; the one who accepts it and sees it as an opportunity to do something more enjoyable remains healthy.

According to "Total Biology of Living Beings", everything has an emotional trigger, like allergies to certain foods, allergies to medications as well as to the environment. I always find it fascinating when someone tells me how their pets and themselves suffer from severe allergies in one area of the country but are doing great in another. The most intriguing part is that the pattern changes for every individual: some people have worse allergies in the desert of Arizona than in a flourishing and humid environment. It makes sense to me that an illness pattern can be related to our deeper life mission: one might need to live in one area versus another in order to fulfill one's life mission. A patient of mine named Stella supports this theory, as she has suffered from a series of unrelated illnesses ever since her family moved to Arizona: this may not be the optimum place for them to fulfill their life missions.

"Total Biology of Living Beings" may have also found a way to explain genetic diseases transmitted from one generation to the next like breast cancer: when a person suffers from a negative emotional response, it initiates a program in the physical body that leads to the illness. This program can then be transmitted to the next generation and replicates by a process called trans-generational memory. One exercise that should be done by everyone, as it can only be beneficial, is to return the emotional baggage to our parents, which was not ours to take in the first place. The simplest example I can give is returning to your mother the fear of flying on an airplane or fear of drowning, if you find that it has prevented you from enjoying flying or swimming. You can write her a letter or else tell her directly. You will be amazed at how much better you will feel inside. If your mother has already transitioned into the next world, you can still use either method. Later, you may want to destroy the written letter, which I believe will bring you immense relief and make you feel much lighter.

Other fascinating research was conducted in Japan by Dr. Masaru Emoto in 2000. He demonstrated that ideas, words, emotions and music had an effect on water molecules: when the energy associated was positive, for example with the words "love", "gratitude" and "thank you", beautiful crystals were formed in the frozen water. When the energy associated was negative, for example with "anger" and "I hate you", ugly crystals were created. Since our body is constituted of seventy percent of water, one has the advantage to fill it with good words, good thoughts and good energy. The same prevails for our pets. This research supports the findings of Rhonda Byrne in her book, *The Secret*, that positive thoughts and words have the powers to heal and attract wealth into our lives.

Additionally, I do believe in the power of names as several pets seem to live up to their names. We should all use caution when we name our best friends. I met a dog named Itchy who ended up with skin problems and was always itchy. Another one named Waters who developed chronic diarrhea. I will always remember a dog named Happy: in spite of an extremely advanced cancer in his abdomen as well as in his anal sac, Happy was focusing on the good in life. Do not tell him that he has cancer, because he does not know it! Happy was just that, happy and acting as normal as can be to everyone's amazement!

CHAPTER 10

Improving conventional medicine

My goal and my hope in writing this book is to open everyone's heart and mind to improve our world and better the lives of all living creatures, one at a time. We can make a difference with every action we take every day. We can all have a positive impact on someone else's life by bringing more joy, hope and healing than we ever thought possible. Together, we can learn to care not only for the physical body, but also for the mind and the soul.

1st idea to improve the care of people and animals worldwide: be human with compassion and communication

In both veterinary and human medicine, there is room for much more compassion. The medical staff often has become used to seeing and performing certain procedures. Building tolerance is normal and imperative to perform the work well and not get emotionally destabilized by the stress of a patient that may be in a critical state. However, every medical staff member must find a healthy balance of sensitivity. Many procedures are done "routinely" and we tend to forget that each patient goes through the procedure only once for the most part, which is therefore not routine to him. Each patient (human or animal) gets scared and anxious and needs support and reassurance from the medical team. Additionally, many of these procedures are painful and remain painful each time that a patient has to go through them.

Improving communication (tearing down the wall) between the medical staff and the patient and his family is also mandatory to better our medical system. Unfortunately, with the incessant increase in law suits, I find that doctors feel pressured to recommend and perform too many diagnostic test options, including referral to specialists, CT scans and MRIs, for almost every single patient, even when common sense, medical knowledge, logic and gut feeling might dictate otherwise. This has led to overfilled emergency rooms, with waiting times ranging from several hours to several months to consult with specialists, costly medical bills, and stressed and overwhelmed patients. If specialists' care was correctly provided according to need and priority, instead of using this "blanket approach", (referred to as justice in the medical ethic code, in regards to distribution of scarce health resources among patients), patients would benefit greatly, medical staff members would not become overworked, they would make fewer mistakes, and the medical system would improve.

It appears that better communication could prevent most law suits from happening by clearing any misunderstandings as soon as they form. In order to achieve adequate communication, I think it is imperative that every medical staff member be passionate about his work. When someone is passionate about his work, love and compassion flow from one's heart to his patients. One becomes more patient, attentive, caring and involved. One takes the time to communicate to his patient what is happening to the physical body, what information each diagnostic test might reveal and what treatment options are available to hopefully regain health.

Additionally, it is imperative that everyone understands that we are all humans, therefore imperfect. We are all here to grow and help each other do the same: we are a team. Apologizing when a mistake is made goes a very long way. Additionally, listening to someone's expression of distress or dismay with the situation will often be all that is needed to make someone feel better. Everyone loves to be told: I hear you; I completely understand how frustrating your situation is; I wish I could do more; I wish I could heal your problem or your pet's problem in the blink of an eye; I wish things were different; I am really sorry that your pet chewed up his stitches; I support you. These words are extremely healing. Be the first one to open the line of communication at any step of the way.

In the medical field, knowledge is constantly changing and evolving, therefore, no one can possibly know everything. As a medical staff member, do not hesitate to tell your patient or his family that you will have to do some research to find an answer. I think patients greatly appreciate honesty. Additionally, the medical team does appreciate when patients tell the truth about what medications they might have taken or what happened that led to an illness. Every detail you share with your medical team is beneficial. The more information that is provided, the better someone can help you. And if you do not know the answer to a question, please simply say: I don't know.

2nd idea to improve the care of people and animals worldwide: treat your patient like your own pet or your own mother

Hold someone's hand or paw. There is always time for a kiss on the forehead or a belly rub. Talk to your patients, animals and humans, and listen to them. Give your patients love and kind words of reassurance. LOVE is always the best treatment.

A smile lights up a room! Can you imagine if *every* nurse, *every* doctor, *every* patient, *every* patient's family members and *every* receptionist smiled at everyone else, even over the phone? A smile is extremely powerful at shifting the energies into positive and healing ones.

Take time to explain to your patient what is going to happen. Several years ago, I developed an unexplained need to talk out loud to my patients before surgery. It made me feel more bonded with them, which gave me confidence for a successful procedure. Now that I have experienced animal communication, I know that animals do feel the energies that we put in our thoughts and words; therefore we should all talk to them, at home and at the hospital.

Feel your words and visualize them too. Animals do understand better when we send them mental pictures. Before a risky procedure, I may ask the pet for his guidance in helping him for the best outcome. Before a rather simple procedure on an elderly pet, I will ask him to stay with us, telling him that he still has several years of great life with his family ahead. If an anesthetized patient is unstable, I will talk to him as well.

I also communicate with my patients to perform radiographs, do a blood draw and other diagnostic tests. First and foremost, with all my respect, I ask my patients permission to perform the diagnostic tests that I believe are needed to help them. I then tell them that it may hurt or be stressful but it will only take a minute if they cooperate. Most cats and dogs understand their names. Each patient should be called by their names and referred to by their names as well. Most dogs already understand the words "lie down", "stay" and "no". I have definitely seen how communication has decreased the need to sedate animals for simple procedures, decreased the need for restraint, and strengthened the bond between teammates, medical staff members and their patients. I would advise medical doctors and nurses to give this technique a try, especially when working with newborns and children. Anesthesiologists, surgeons and emergency staff members should also use this method when helping unconscious patients.

3rd idea to improve the care of people and animals worldwide: work as a team and make sure your team works

One of the most important factors to promote healing is that the patient and his family are comfortable being themselves around their medical team. Everyone has unique needs and personal beliefs. Make sure your team inspires you to be yourself and motivates you to share your needs and beliefs. If a patient needs to ask for her deceased grandmother's guidance during her surgery, she should have the opportunity and support to do so. The medical team should put all the odds in their favor for a smooth and successful procedure and recovery. I have assisted with several rituals with families during euthanasia ceremonies and I always find them fascinating. Although there are some that I can not relate to, I can tell how healing they are for the families, and therefore, I always give them my unconditional support. No one should judge any technique that brings healing and peace to someone else.

A patient, his family and his medical team must connect and

work together towards a common goal: healing. Their energies must flow in the same direction. Set yourself up for success as a doctor or as a patient. If you feel uncomfortable in a certain situation, make the necessary changes right away. Although most people should get along with proper communication and human skills, we all vibrate on different levels and our energies will sometimes clash. I have come to the conclusion that no one can help everyone and similarly, no one can be helped by everyone either. Listen to your feelings and inner voice.

Additionally, if a surgery is scheduled but you are suddenly having the worst feeling about it, cancel it as suggested by the neurosurgeon Dr. Allan Hamilton in his book *The Scalpel and the Soul*. Be involved in your own healing and in your pet's healing. Don't be a victim, be a leader.

4th idea to improve the care of people and animals worldwide: be actively involved in your own healing and in the healing of your pet

The main benefits of conventional medicine are to stabilize the physical body during times of crisis (asthma, stroke, trauma, infection). Conventional medicine buys time and brings rapid relief to both people and animals. Unfortunately, we all know that conventional medicine can not help everyone in all situations. Sometimes, conventional doctors must tell their patients that there is nothing they can do for their disease. You then must decide where to go from there. In such cases, the doctor might be right that no treatment modality will help you. However, there might be other ways to help yourself, which is certainly worth investigating. I have two very close geriatric feline friends who have rallied more times than ever expected. No one knows for sure when our time is up. I think it is wise for everyone to become actively involved in their healing as well as in the healing of their pets, and not "wait" for someone to magically heal their ailments.

A diagnosis is a label. Everyone will express the disease differently. Instead of feeling shattered by it, see a diagnosis as an opportunity to grow. Choose to embrace it and learn from it. Research all your options and make your decision. My dear friend, Brigid, called me when her canine friend Coco was battling cancer. Coco was in remission from his cancer but Brigid kept hearing the words from her veterinarian: "the cancer will come back". Based on published studies, the medical community does have an idea of how long most patients live once they are diagnosed with a certain disease. However, no one can predict someone's longevity in any given case. No one can say for sure that Coco will get sick again or when he will. Each situation is very unique. Coco is sharing this experience with Brigid. No one else can possibly have the exact same emotions, personalities, past life experiences and current life missions that have led to this disease. It is important to accept that what is happening is part of a bigger plan and is intended for growth of the souls involved. Success is not calculated by whether the patient cures the disease and survives. To the contrary, success is calculated by how much growing we do, how much love and support we share, and by being fair to the patient in the way we care for him, doing what he wants us to do for him. Each patient with cancer has different needs and wants.

Aside from conventional medicine, there are several other tools that can help one heal, which can all be included under the name of alternative medicine. These different methods of restoring health focus mainly on long-term health maintenance as well as prevention of illnesses. Some examples of alternative medicine therapies are naturopathy, Chinese medicine, herbal and homeopathic remedies, chiropractics, acupuncture, total biology of living beings, applied kinesiology, hypnosis, energy work, psychic work, aromatherapy and music therapy. I deeply believe that no one tool can help everybody in every situation. We should therefore investigate and pick the necessary tools for healing to occur.

Integrative medicine is a groundbreaking concept well developed by Andrew Weil, M.D. over the last decade. Integrative medicine is a healing-oriented medicine that combines both approaches, conventional and alternative medicine. It takes into consideration the whole person (body, mind and spirit) with emphasis on prevention and lifestyle, such as nutrition, exercise and stress reduction. Dr. Weil's work has opened the door to using a combination of healing methods, whatever works, to heal an ailment in a specific patient.

My life experiences have taught me that not all patients suffering from the same condition will respond the same way to therapies, whether conventional or alternative. Again, based on what emotion might have triggered the illness in the first place, or what the illness is here to teach, in relation to one's life purpose, the speed in healing, recovery and recurrence will vary greatly. If the illness comes from a negative emotion, once the mind shifts, the body can shift as well, inhibiting the progression of a disease, or else healing a disease that was labeled incurable. My husband's friend, Tulia, was diagnosed with end-stage lymphoma and the medical community had run out of options to help her. She was given only a couple of months to live. She went home and miraculously lived for another forty years. The cancer completely left her body. Miracles do exist.

This brings us to a discussion of the concept of Intuitive Medicine. A medical intuitive is an alternative medicine practitioner who uses his intuitive abilities to find the cause of a physical or emotional condition. A patient trying to figure out why he got sick and how to prevent it from happening again is where intuitive medicine begins. Animal communication and psychic work performed with the goal of healing is also intuitive medicine.

I was thrilled to learn about the *Academy of Intuition Medicine*® in California, founded in 1984. It is a globally recognized academic school for those interested in developing their natural intuitive abilities to pursue a career as a professional medical intuitive, to integrate intuitive abilities into a current career, or simply to improve their personal lives.

Again, be involved in your own healing. Participate as much as you can. Read about your diagnosis and your prescribed medications. Be aware of how the medication works and what side effects to look for. Do some soul searching to find out the cause of your illness or of your pet's illness. Analyze the options given to you by any of the professionals you are seeking help from and make sure to pick the option that is the most in tune with how you feel. Waiting around for a magic cure or else trusting blindly can only lead to hurt and disappointment.

When I broke my thumb, I did not want anyone else near me but a surgeon. When I needed to understand the reasons for a low-grade asthma that I had for several years, I reached for intuitive medicine. To speed up my recovery from a cold, I boost my immune system with alternative medicine. Every type of healing has its place and plays an important role in the team.

5th idea to improve the care of people and animals worldwide: treat the patient not the disease

One particular situation that is a regular source of frustration for pet owners in veterinary hospitals is the care of their elderly pet. Of course we could, once again, perform all the diagnostic tests in the book on every senior citizen, whether human or animal. Is this truly the purpose of the medical system? Granted, as we get older, things tend to fall apart: degenerative joint disease, heart disease, renal disease, etc. Do we have to intervene all the time? Especially when several diseases that occur in elderly patients can never be completely cured. Are we truly helping by intervening or are we harming? I believe the number one goal of medicine should be to focus on giving patients as much quality of life as possible, with or without medications. We can help a feline friend live significantly longer by flushing his kidneys with either subcutaneously fluids or even hospitalization for a few days. Is this being fair to this animal? Only he will give us the answer. I do wish a good life for all my patients, my family, my friends and myself, with as little pain and stress as possible, with as much happiness as possible, for as long as possible. However, the duration of one's life is the least important of the factors listed. In other words, who wants to live forever, if there is no happiness, and if there is constant pain and stress?

From what I have seen, medical students are taught to do everything they can to keep the patient alive, by treating the disease. Veterinary students are also taught to treat the disease, however, with animals, there is the additional option of euthanasia. The way I practice medicine today is very different from when I first graduated from veterinary school ten years ago. The School of Life has taught me an important lesson: suffering is worse than dying. When I first graduated, I recommended that all owners of elderly cats in chronic renal failure give their cats subcutaneous injections of fluids at home, or possibly even hospitalize them for a few days, combined with an array of oral medications (for which several owners had to literally chase their cats around the house to catch them, twice daily!). The conversation about stress, quality of life and dignity was nonexistent. I am sure some owners only followed my recommendations due to my enthusiasm of believing that I was doing the right thing. I am sure some of these owners were torn between my recommendations and their hearts telling them not to cause additional stress and pain to their elderly pets. There is a fine line between treatment and torture. Today, I always weigh all options with all clients for all patients. One of these options includes doing nothing. The right answer is given by the patient. Some cats will allow us to medicate them and poke them with a needle everyday, whereas some others will not. If one cat is still feeling great without symptoms of renal failure and the owner has already declined intervention, my recommendation is then to forget that he has a "diagnosis". Enjoy each day with your pet, share as much love as possible, until symptoms start occurring. When your best friend tells you it is time to free him from his suffering, honor his wishes. Honoring our loved ones' requests, being fair to them and preserving their dignity is by far the priority in making medical decisions.

I would like to discuss the notion of common sense, a notion that I was very fortunate to learn during my training with one particular specialist. I believe practitioners should use common sense in any decision they make. No matter what the book says or what the teacher says, ask yourself, "Does this make sense for my patient and his situation?" Too many times I have to face situations where theory and real life are in discordance. Of course the right answer is what your common sense dictates. For example, when wanting to hospitalize a patient who gets extremely anxious away from his family, the pros and cons of being hospitalized must be weighed and communicated adequately with the family. Everyone appreciates having their own emotional needs as well as their pets' emotional needs cared for along with their physical bodies. These two are so closely related in fact, that many patients will not return to normal health until they are returned to the comfort of home, in a stress-free environment. My recommendation is to hospitalize a patient only if home care is judged inadequate. This means that the benefits of being hospitalized (with intensive nursing care given by professionals, specialized equipments to monitor the patient and administer medications) must outweigh the stress caused by being away from home. Additionally, I keep the patient in the hospital for as little time as is needed, and return him home as quickly as possible.

I will share with you the story of Buster, which reinforces many important points: the first one is that allowing two and four-legged family members to visit a sick patient is extremely beneficial to healing. Who would not want the support and reassurance of a brother or mother when they are sick? Who would not want their cat, dog, horse or bird to come cuddle up with them when they are not feeling well? A patient, particularly a sick child or an animal, can easily believe they have been abandoned when they are taken away from their family for a prolonged period of time. This was the case of Buster. Buster is a family dog that was hospitalized for severe pancreatitis. After a few days, although he had stopped vomiting, he was still not interested in eating and looked very depressed. He had the energy to get up and walk outside, however something was wrong. Talking to mom over the phone about his questionable progress, I decided to have his family visit. When Buster saw them, he began climbing the walls of his kennel and barking with enthusiasm. His family had truly brought him out of his depressive state. It became clear that Buster thought he had been abandoned. Knowing that his family loved him gave him hope and strength to continue fighting and healing.

Because he did not want to eat even in the presence of his family, we decided to keep him hospitalized on intravenous fluids for one more night. However, Buster had another plan in mind. As soon as his family left the hospital, he began howling, jumping in his kennel and within an hour he had chewed off his intravenous catheter. His message was clear: "I am feeling better and it is time for me to go home." His family and I agreed to send him home immediately in the hopes that he would start eating in a comfortable environment, which he did. Supported by mom and dad's love and care, Buster recovered fully and quickly!

To reinforce the importance of focusing on quality of life of a patient at all times, I would like to discuss another situation where friction frequently occurs between pet owners and veterinary hospitals. Regularly, we meet elderly dogs with such severe pain from arthritis that they can not skip one dose of their pain medication. The family understands that performing blood tests at regular intervals to evaluate their pet's kidney and liver function is extremely beneficial in quickly identifying possible side effects from the pain medication. Some medications are better tolerated by some individuals than others and performing blood tests is helpful in picking the safest medication to spare the kidneys and liver. However, this is another example where theory differs from real life. Someone's finances may prevent them from being able to keep repeating those tests. Alternatively, some pets, especially at an advanced age, may build an extreme amount of stress which makes performing a blood draw a risky procedure. It only makes sense that the priority should be for the owner to continue to have access to the pain medication that his best friend desperately needs, whether or not blood tests are performed. When someone expresses a difficulty in following recommendations, proper communication will lead to a compromise that benefits everyone: the pet, the family and the medical team. A waiver can be required to be signed by the patient and his family, stating that one declines performing blood tests and understands the risks involved. Everybody wins in this situation. When a client becomes upset, ask yourself, "Was I right in my doings? How could I have helped this patient and his family better? Where did we miscommunicate and misunderstand each other? How can I still help?"

The other aspect of treating the patient and not the disease comes in play when elderly patients have curable diseases. I will always remember two pets in particular who taught me, early on in my career, an important lesson; that although getting old is often not easy for the physical body, age itself is not a disease. Foxy was an eighteen-year-old Pomeranian with severe gastroenteritis. Although her dad knew that it could be the end of her life, he was willing to try something. Due to her extreme stress level away from dad, hospitalization was not an option. For several days, dad would bring her in to receive fluids under her skin to prevent dehydration from her vomiting and diarrhea. She was on oral medications to soothe her gastrointestinal tract. Although it took longer than average for her to get over her illness, I did not want to give up. Foxy was a determined little girl, full of spunk and looked like she wanted to live, and she did.

Frankie was a fourteen-year-old English pointer with liver disease. His skin had turned completely yellow, which indicated severe illness. His febrile state combined with his blood analysis made me suspect an acute bacterial infection. Due to his age, his owners had declined extraordinary measures, however, they finally allowed me to hospitalize him for intravenous fluids and antibiotics. Frankie, just like Foxy, looked like he was not ready to give up. I could just feel in my heart that I had to give him a chance to live. Frankie responded quickly to medications, returned home after three days and lived a couple more years.

I believe that specialization in medicine has brought a lot of good to better understand, diagnose and treat diseases. It only makes sense that when someone focuses on one aspect of the physical body, one's medical knowledge and proficiency increase in helping that part of the body. However, every specialist must still remember to treat the patient, not the disease. It is very unfortunate when an oncologist recommends chemotherapy to help the cancer of an elderly patient, who is also blind and can barely walk from severe arthritis. What is the overall quality of life? I do admire a surgeon who does not recommend surgery on every patient. How can a child in a coma be kept on artificial life support when she is battling cancer (which the oncologist is looking after) and congestive heart failure (which the cardiologist is looking after)? Who is in charge of caring for the whole patient? What are the chances that we will cure this child or give her any kind of quality of life? Luckily for this one child, a caring pediatrician remembered fairness to her patient and was able to convince her parents to facilitate her transition into the next world and free her from her suffering.

6th idea to improve the care of people and animals worldwide: remember that quality of death is as important as quality of life

Once one reaches the point where quality of life is no longer possible, I believe the focus must change to quality of death. When treatment truly becomes synonymous with torture, something must change. Again, every patient is unique and every situation is different. We did perform surgery on our pet Hayley when she was thirteen years old to repair a ruptured cruciate ligament in one of her knees. Assessing her overall condition, aside from being unable to use her injured leg from an acute trauma, she was doing beautifully and her arthritis was very minimal. Hayley's quality of life was suddenly extremely poor due to her injured knee, which we knew surgery could fix, and it did. Within two days, she was already putting weight on her leg, and after ten days, she was back to normal. By performing surgery, we bought her almost a full year of great quality of life.

When my college basketball coach, Ghyslain, was diagnosed with stomach cancer, it was a different story. He tried chemotherapy but knew right away that it was not for him. He chose a shorter survival time, but with a better quality of life. During his last three months, he did everything he wished to do and even planned his own funeral. He had a very peaceful passing, in the comfort of home, feeling supported, loved and guided by his girlfriend, the love of his life. She selflessly gave him the strength and courage to free himself, although it meant leaving her. Together, they experienced the most magnificent voyage. She gave him dignity and peace, which is truly the best gift anyone can receive.

Another heartwarming story is the one of a dear client of mine, Mr. Stinner. Mr. Stinner was a wonderful man, who spent his life rescuing as many dogs as he could. He wished the world could have been a kinder place for everyone. After many years of battling different illnesses, he finally reached a point where his quality of life was very poor and his suffering had become unbearable. Worried about leaving his wife of many years, he shared with her his concerns of leaving her but also his need to find peace and free himself. As soon as his extremely loving and selfless wife gave him permission to leave her, he was able to transition peacefully within only a few days. Although it hurts to lose a loved one, knowing that our loved one is at peace and pain free brings extreme comfort.

7th idea to improve the care of people and animals worldwide: remember that we are all going to die one day, do not miss your exit door

Most people are afraid of the truth but it remains the truth: we are all going to die. What is less sure is with how much dignity and how much suffering. Everyone can only hope to have a peaceful transition, for themselves and their loved ones, with as much dignity and as little suffering as possible. Several books written by mediums talk about the concept of exit doors: every soul has five possible exit doors throughout life. These are the only times where a soul can exit the physical body and return Home. This concept can definitely explain those situations when someone dies of a minor incident whereas someone else survives a catastrophic situation.

Just like animals, people develop strong emotional bonds that can make it difficult for them to let go, therefore prolonging suffering. It is imperative for these ties to be broken. Additionally, to facilitate our transition, we must complete any unfinished business as well as clear any worries that we may have. My limited experience with people at the end of their lives has been that again, personality matters. Some people will sacrifice themselves for their loved ones and "allow" the medical team to perform one more surgery to buy their family time to say goodbye when unfortunately, they are ready to transition and should let go for their own sake. By sacrificing themselves, some people miss their exit door, remaining in their physical body which is only continuing to deteriorate further, experiencing suffering that could have been avoided. It is heart wrenching to see a loved one suffer powerlessly and I wish more people would be able to selflessly allow their suffering loved ones to transition quickly when the opportunity presents itself, even when the family staying behind is not quite ready. No one is ever ready to say goodbye to a loved one. I will always admire my dear friend Pam for finding the strength to be selfless and allow her gravely ill son to return Home at a very young age. She obeyed his wishes. I know how grateful he is for having had a mom who understood his needs.

I believe the animal model can be used to assess our own quality of life, or the one of a family member or friend: Is my loved one in pain? Is he eating and drinking normally? Is he able to go to the bathroom without soiling himself? Is he doing his favorite things as he used to? Does he still have enthusiasm and interest for favorite toys, treats and family members? Is he able to go on walks, get up without assistance? Is he having more bad days than good days? How much dignity does my loved one have left? Is he trying to tell me: "I need your help, it's time, I can't do this any longer" OR "I'm ok, I'd like to stay a little longer"?

If the decision is made for yourself or your loved one that quality of life can not be reached, it is time to focus on quality of death.

Discuss with your medical doctor ways of decreasing suffering and easing the transition process. Trust your heart and your inner feelings. Take it one day at a time. When you are helping someone make a difficult decision like undergoing life-threatening surgery or cancer therapy, weigh the pros and cons of each option. Listen to your loved one's needs and put yourself in his shoes, just like you would to help an animal. Ask your loved one how he feels deep inside. Did he receive any "signs of guidance" that can help him make the decision of undergoing surgery or not? Doing chemotherapy or not? Sort out all the feelings involved to ease the decision making process: what do I want for myself, what does my loved one want and need? Being selfless is not easy but is mandatory, as our loved one's needs must precede our needs. Just like we do for animals, give permission to your loved one to go when the time comes, therefore minimizing his struggle. Tell him that you wish he would stay with you for many more years but leave it up to him. As hard as it will be to be separated for a while, he has to do what is best for him and go back Home when Home is calling. Thank him for all the good times together. He has been such a wonderful companion and you will always love him.

Somewhere inside, I think that everybody has the ability to transition peacefully and naturally once their life mission is completed, by sorting out their emotions adequately. Giving permission to our loved ones to follow their life plan and leave us when their time has come is extremely powerful in facilitating their transition. Of course, having recourse to euthanasia to free our loved ones from their suffering would ease this process as well. I deeply believe that suffering is worse than dying. I hope we can use the animal model to rebuild a caring medical system for ourselves.

All mediums on my path have agreed with me: some people's physical bodies have become too deteriorated and their minds are too far gone for any more growing of the soul to happen. Only suffering is left. Some people's souls have even left their bodies, and yet remain connected to them, unfortunately hanging between two worlds, while the physical body is still alive, in a sad state of deterioration. Seeing how much peace euthanasia brings to animals and their families, how can we not wish the same for ourselves and our human loved ones?

Several months ago, I felt strongly attracted to visit the butterfly exhibit at the botanical gardens. This experience allowed me to truly reflect on the cycle of life, which we are all a part of. I learned that many butterflies live only one month. The exhibit had butterflies of all ages: young ones, full of life, flying fast and racing playfully with one another; adults, more mature, taking a nice smooth flight and landing on visitors' shoulders, laps and hands. I saw a gentleman with a gorgeous friend on his shoulder. He looked at me and said, "Look, you have one too!" I then found the older butterflies, full of wisdom, lying on the large window sill. Some would try in vain to fly as their wings had become fragile and frail. Some others had already accepted their "senior" status and were quietly waiting for their time of transition. The euthanasia question popped up again in my head, who should we euthanize? Which butterflies are suffering? How about people? I think the right answer is: nature intended us to experience all the different stages of the cycle of life. It is okay to be old, it is okay not to be able to play sports anymore, and it is okay to need assistance getting in and out of the car, as long as there is still quality of life. Euthanasia is not for the old ones but for the sick ones of any age, when a cure is not possible and suffering must stop. That made sense to me, for all living creatures.

How do we assess quality of life? Through the series of questions listed before, and ultimately, through the heart of the living creature involved as well as his loved ones' selfless hearts. Mediums, intuitives, shamans and energy workers are extremely beneficial to help as well. What does this creature want? Have we reached an exit door? The butterfly exhibit guide in the main room must have sensed my troubles as I was sadly staring at the older ones with broken wings. He instructed me to go see the butterflies in the birthing room. When I arrived, all I could see were rows and rows of cocoons. Then I spotted a first full grown butterfly hanging from his cocoon, then another one. Then I found one that had his wings stuck together all shriveled up and wet as he had just dropped out of his cocoon. Finally, my eyes locked with one moving cocoon and I assisted in the birth of a butterfly! How beautiful! It will take a while before he is ready to see the world as he must dry and spread out these magnificent wings first. I was so excited for him! Live to the fullest, especially when you are a butterfly, because a month is quickly over. This reminded me of how I had to live too, adding to the latest life lessons of playing more and having fun before I become a senior creature on the window sill. All the stages of the cycle of life are as valuable. One needs to spend time experiencing and enjoying each one of them.

8th idea to improve the care of people and animals worldwide: allow all family members to say goodbye to their departed loved one to find closure and peace

Again, animals grieve like we do. Just like people need to know when a loved one has transitioned, human or animal, so do animals. It brings so much peace, understanding and closure to an animal to visit with the deceased body of a human or animal friend. Animals must be able to say goodbye too. When someone transitions, human or animal, at the hospital for example, it is mandatory for the remaining pets to be brought to visit with the body, or else to bring the body home for everyone to understand. It eases their grieving process tremendously, bringing them peace and closure, and allowing them to return much faster to their daily routine and activities. This can not be emphasized enough.

The concept of moving on is easy to evaluate in people who lose a dear friend, human or animal. In my experiences, the people who move on the fastest are the ones who can process their emotions the fastest. People who have listened to their own needs at each step of the way, asked questions, followed their heart, performed this or that diagnostic test, tried this or that treatment option, who knew when to switch their focus from quality of life to quality of death, people who have no regrets, who are at peace inside and genuinely feel happy for their departed friend, are the ones who move on the easiest and the fastest. On the other end, it can be extremely difficult for someone to ever get over the loss of a loved one if regrets are present. When this happens, one can only take it one step at a time and work through each regret, finding a way to heal every single emotion and find peace again. This may mean writing a letter to a departed loved one, expressing everything you wish you had said to him or everything you wish you had done differently. Remember that we are all here to grow. This journey of growing and learning lessons can sometimes be painful. However, our departed loved one never holds a grudge and only wants for us to feel at peace inside.

In spite of the emotional trauma caused by saying goodbye to a loved one, and the initial feelings of never wanting to adopt another pet or make new friends from fear of having to go through the same difficult process, everyone agrees that human and animal friendship is what makes life fun! People and animals often walk in our lives without us even searching. For some families, it only takes a few weeks, even only days, before they bring their new four-legged best friend to me to meet and examine. A new best friend in someone's life is like a breath of fresh air. We must live in the now and enjoy the beauty of life!

9th idea to improve the care of people and animals worldwide: the best Doctor is someone who remembers how it feels to be a patient

The first principle of medicine is: DO NO HARM. I would like to continue this principle with "…to the physical body and the emotional body, therefore, be careful and gentle." After Hayley transitioned, my motto became: be fair to pets. Hayley was the best patient. She would let us do anything we needed to do to her, although we could tell it was stressful for her. Since she transitioned, when I take care of an animal, I can hear her say: "Be gentle, it is stressful to be a patient but I trust you."

It all starts in school. Medical students, nurses and assistants (in both veterinary and human medicine) need to be taught how to use needles gently, to ask permission from their patients (human and animal), and to respect their patients. They need to realize the stress and pain that their patients are going through while patiently waiting for the students to be successful at their first blood draw and catheter placement. Students must be grateful and say "thank you" to all their patients for allowing them to learn these new skills.

We do not decide what is stressful for someone else; listen to what your patient tells you. You can not tell your patient that his fear is unjustified. Everyone decides how much they can physically and emotionally handle. Going to the dentist uses up an extreme amount of my energy. Losing my baby teeth as a child was one of the worst times of my life. Although you can try to convince pets and people that something is fun, everyone has a unique perception that can be very difficult to change. While I wish I was as courageous as my cousin who I saw having fun twisting each of her teeth until they fell off, for me, each loose tooth became a stressful and never ending journey as I could not bring myself to touch it, let alone pull it.

Again, for each patient there will be a unique treatment. Find what is in each pet's best interest, what is the safest, what brings the lowest stress level. Tailor your care based on the patient's personality, emotional needs, lifestyle, relationship with his family (how much the family can help him), the role that the pet plays in his family's life, and the patient's soul mission.

Use an ear thermometer to take the animal's temperature. The most accurate one that I have found and that I use for animals is the Braun thermoscan ear thermometer designed for humans. If you have to struggle with an animal for five minutes to be successful at taking his temperature, it will be elevated from the stress and the struggle the animal just went through. An animal who can wrestle you that badly is not running a fever. Use your common sense and know when to stop. Always remember what you are trying to accomplish and is it worth the stress? Why are we trying to perform this procedure? Is there a better way, an easier way that would work better for all? The family and the medical team must work together at minimizing the stress and fear level for the animal. Sometimes, this does require being creative. My husband is the one who has successfully created a unique nail trim protocol for our dog, which only he can successfully perform as Yogi trusts him and him only. After a couple of years of training, positive reinforcement, "Whale Done" methods and animal communication, we have also successfully taught Yogi to remain calm when he gets a cactus needle stuck in his paw or on his face to allow us to remove it. Yogi has sure taught us patience, perseverance, to be creative, to remember to make a procedure fun and to give lots of praises when he is a good boy. We could not be more proud of him!

I wish all families could be as involved as possible with their pet's care, especially with grooming, nail trimming and toothbrushing. Several procedures can be taught and learned. We all feel safer when our loved ones perform the stressful procedures. Additionally, the family members have more time on their hands to be patient and attentive to their pets' needs, therefore making a stressful procedure as enjoyable as possible for their pets. Learn to do as much as you can. Keep the routine so your pet knows what is coming. The same person should perform specific procedures. One should not perform a procedure if one is uncomfortable and should ask to be taught first. A bad experience will be difficult to correct, for example with nail trimming. It hurts to have a nail trimmed too short (and bleed). Your pet may become scared of having his feet ever touched again. Care must be taken to avoid such a costly mistake. About cats, most cats never need to be bathed. Cats are such clean animals, they clean themselves regularly and getting a bath is extremely stressful to them.

There are some medical procedures that can be performed in various ways, and it is best to choose the procedural method that induces the least stress to the animal. One of the best examples I have to illustrate this are the different procedures used to obtain urine for a urinalysis. Too many families and medical staff members decide, to save time and hassle, to get a urine sample by performing a cystocentesis on the animal. This procedure involves inserting a needle through the abdominal wall and into the bladder of the animal, which is awake but restrained, to collect urine into a syringe. What are other ways to obtain a urine sample? Other ways that are also stressful in my experience are via catheterization or manual expression. The way I prefer by far is the free catch method: the owner collects urine at home when the dog urinates, by catching it before it touches the ground. Alternatively, a medical staff member can help you accomplish this by following you outside the hospital with your pet. I have a client who taught his dog to urinate on command, how wonderful! For cats, fill the litter box with beads, rocks, beans, hydrophobic sand litter or else plastic litter, which allows collection of the urine from the box.

Why try to avoid a cystocentesis? The first reason is because it is a stressful and painful procedure for the patient. Secondly, it is traumatic to the body and risks of rupturing the bladder are inherent. I have performed cystocentesis on anesthetized patients during surgery and many times I have seen large bruises forming on the bladder wall from the needle puncturing a blood vessel on its way. Because one has no control over avoiding such blood vessels, urine samples collected by cystocentesis are often contaminated with blood which makes interpretation very difficult. When blood is found in a urine sample obtained by free catch or in the litter box, it is much more indicative of a disease being present. The rare occasions when a cystocentesis is warranted are to differentiate a bladder infection from a lower urinary tract disease (like vaginitis or prostatitis), or when a urine sample must be cultured for bacterial identification.

I wish all pet owners would realize what they are putting their pets through just for their own convenience of not having to do the work at home. The same concept applies to allowing a medical staff member to retrieve a fecal sample by using a rectal probe when the pet owner can easily bring a fresh sample given by his pet everyday. How do you want to be cared for as a patient? I believe everyone wants comfort, safety and as little stress and trauma as possible. Ask to be present with your pet when he gets his nails trimmed or blood drawn. Insist that the medical staff member shaves the hair to access the vein more easily, decreasing stress and trauma during the blood draw. Ask the medical team how your pet did when dropped off for surgery. Again, know what you are putting your pet through. Animals, like us, remember bad experiences and can remain scared and scarred for the rest of their lives.

If we determined that one method does not work, we find a better one. We finally figured out that the best way for Pete to have his nails trimmed and his blood drawn was when his dad held him against his chest, with a muzzle on, his feet dangling in the air, while mom rubbed his head. Additionally, we found that if Pete waited outdoors until the medical team was completely ready it helped greatly. Although Pete does not seem to mind which staff member is performing the procedure, some others like Kaibab seemed to respond favorably to a female doctor accompanied by a specific technician. Every time, we try to repeat the procedure identically so the pet knows what is going to happen, therefore decreasing his stress level as much as we possibly can.

Knowing when to use sedatives to decrease the stress of performing simple procedures on animals is very important. One drug that is by far underutilized in the veterinary field in my opinion is Telazol. Its main advantage is that it can be given in a very small dose and easily injected under the skin, in the muscle or intravenously.

Combined with other commonly used sedatives, Telazol is wonderful to care for feral cats or other very anxious animals.

Sedatives should always be used when a patient clearly demonstrates a high level of stress and fear. There is no room for ego in medicine, when trying to win some kind of battle with a feral cat or any other aggressive animal will only lead to someone getting hurt, you or the animal. Respect aggressive pets and allow them to be scared of what you are trying to do to them. Send them your love, support and understanding. Be creative in finding ways to comfort these pets.

10th idea to improve the care of people and animals worldwide: consider adopting a soul in need of a good home (animal or human) instead of reproducing

Due to the severe pet overpopulation crisis that the world is going through, it has become a growing source of frustration among veterinary hospitals to find unaltered pets whose families refuse to spay or neuter. However, we must all remember that breeding itself is not the problem, as it can actually be a rich experience for children to participate in raising kittens and puppies. The problem comes when everyone does it, in a disorganized or unplanned way. We end up with several unwanted puppies and kittens worldwide that are abandoned in the streets or else in overcrowded shelters. In the past years, up to five million healthy dogs and cats had to be euthanized every year in the United States due to the pet overpopulation problem.

Comparing this sad situation with the human situation, the problem is the same: overpopulation. The reason for it is the same: uncontrolled and unplanned breeding. The orphanages are overfilled and several other unfortunate children growing up in dysfunctional families will become homeless at a very young age.

The ethical question that presents itself becomes: how to fix this problem of overpopulation for both animals and people? Unfortunately, there is no easy answer. For animals in the developed countries, we are already promoting and performing all of the options: sterilization (surgical removal of reproductive organs – a great tip for veterinarians: keeping the front legs loose while sterilizing a female helps tremendously!), education to prevent breeding, and interruption of pregnancy (abortion). However, it appears that it will be a long lasting battle that may never be won.

In people, the possible options to decrease overpopulation fuel highly agitated debates. Probably the one aspect that most people currently agree on is the fact that the planet is becoming quickly overwhelmed by too many people. We are using up its resources at an alarming rate. One way to help fix the problem is truly by improving our education of children at a young age, at home and in school. Unfortunately, no one is perfect. In spite of the best education and the best prevention, mistakes do happen.

For animals, the scientific community has proven the huge benefits of sterilization, not only as a means to reduce overpopulation but also in improving health: drastic decrease in rate of breast cancer, prostatic diseases, aggression and behavioral problems. The combination of sterilization and abortion is also performed routinely, especially in shelters, when it is judged that the puppies or kittens will have a difficult life, most likely a life in a shelter as no one will ever adopt them, or else will end up being abandoned in the streets. It is not something that we enjoy doing, however, I believe that all veterinarians feel relieved to save these puppies and kittens from the difficult lives they would have lived if born unwanted and uncared for. There are enough animals currently in that situation that we are trying to help.

In 2001, more than two million unmarried women had an unplanned pregnancy. Following the animal model, when the situation presents itself with a dark future for a child to be raised in a dysfunctional family, without the appropriate support and love, where the parents see the child as a burden and feel resentment towards him, abortion is in my eyes the kindest gift to give this soul.

Every situation is unique and the decision must come from the heart of the mother. What quality of life will my child have? What quality of life will I have? Can I provide him with a safe, loving and caring environment? Am I emotionally able to care for a child? Am I barely able to care for myself, therefore, it would be in the soul's best interest to return Home and come back later when I am ready? Can I live with the decision of keeping him? Can I live with the decision of returning him to the spirit world? What will be the long-term impact on my life? Again, no one is perfect and everybody makes mistakes. We are all here to grow and abortion can be a healing and growing experience when done at the right time and under the right circumstances.

For both species, humans and animals, please strongly consider adopting a soul in need of a good home instead of reproducing.

11th idea to improve the care of people and animals worldwide: say no to cosmetic surgeries and convenience surgeries

I will first discuss cosmetic surgeries, which in theory will make you and your pet look better. I believe everyone should feel good about themselves and the way they look, however, I find that our modern society has taken it too far. Remember that animals do not care about how they look. Furthermore, anesthesia is never safe and should never be used unless the benefits outweigh the risks, for both our pets and us. You may not see the negative effects of anesthesia on the body for several years to come, but they are there, even with the most sophisticated machines in human medicine, our body is still ingesting foreign substances that affect all the cells in our body.

In veterinary medicine, although more and more hospitals are doing a great job of using the safest anesthetic techniques on your pet, there are still too many that cut major corners. Again, these pets may wake up from anesthesia normally, however, they may end up in liver or kidney failure only a few months following the anesthesia, which I have seen happen when people had opted for a cheaper surgery. Please ask pertinent questions of your veterinary team in order to make sure that your pet is safe. To insure safety, you should get a yes answer to the following questions: Will my pet be given gas anesthesia? Will he have an intravenous catheter and fluids running through his body? Will his blood pressure be checked every five minutes? Will my pet be given oxygen via an endotracheal tube? Will my pet have blood tests before surgery? Will his body temperature be checked regularly? Will my pet receive medication to relieve pain? Will the surgery be done in a sterile way? Does the staff member performing anesthesia know how to evaluate my pet for anesthetic dept (blink reflex, jaw tone, elevation of third eyelid, eye position, heart rate, respiratory rate, blood pressure)?

How much stress do you really want to go through or put your pet through? If the cosmetic surgery is for your pet, I can guarantee you that a surgery is never pleasurable. Again, pets do not care about their look. To them, all they get out of a cosmetic surgery like an ear crop is pain and stress. Please be fair to your pet and don't do it.

The other cosmetic surgery that should be banned in my opinion is dewclaw removal and tail docking in awake, newborn puppies. One may say that the puppies will forget the pain and stress they suffered from quickly, however, I have seen puppies dying immediately following the procedure. Why does our society agree to torture dogs to follow breed standards? This procedure is extremely stressful, painful and purely cosmetic. Remember the emotional trauma that the soul experiences as well as the repercussion on its mental and physical health.

The biggest convenience surgeries in pets are de-barking in dogs and de-clawing in cats. Unfortunately, convenience means "done to make the owner feel better, not to make the pet feel better". What if it were you? How would you feel? Are we being fair to these animals? Is this how nature intended it? Are these procedures morally okay to do? I completely understand that a constantly barking dog is annoying, as is a cat who scratches the furniture. What is this pet trying to tell us? Can we see this experience as an opportunity to grow together?

The de-barking procedure is sickening to watch and causes permanent scarring of the trachea (windpipe through which we all breathe) that can be severe enough to make further intubation impossible when a life-saving surgery becomes needed. I believe that if the pet owner saw the procedure done, it would convince him not to do it.

I hope we can all open our hearts and listen to our animals when they are trying to teach us something. It does take patience and perseverance, maybe a change in lifestyle and consultation with a pet trainer, veterinarian or animal communicator. In any cases, surgery is not the answer in my opinion.

A cat needs his claws. Scratching is a normal feline behavior. Although scratching does serve to shorten and condition the claws, the primary reasons that cats scratch are to mark their territory and to stretch. Stretching is essential for the health of all muscles, bones and tendons of the body. Cats also use their claws to grasp toys, hold objects and food, groom and scratch themselves, climb and walk, and lastly defend themselves. Cats can only walk normally if they have all their claws.

Removing a cat's claws severely "handicaps" him in all aspects of his life. It causes serious and irreversible emotional, psychological and physical damage. Declawed cats (which means they had surgical amputations of all the first bones of their toes, which hold the claws) experience unnecessary stress, fear, pain and anxiety that often lead to decreased self-confidence, increased aggression, development of behavioral and/or physical problems (reluctance to use the litter box, chronic limping).

Seventy percent of cats being brought to shelters for behavioral problems are declawed. On February 8th, 2010, there were 5401 declawed cats in shelters in USA/Canada waiting hopelessly for a good home. If you do not have the patience or time to guide a cat on how to use their claws in your home, please do not adopt one.

The last convenience procedure that I will discuss is convenience euthanasia. Although the world is overpopulated, I find it very sad that healthy and loving animals, or animals with curable diseases, are being euthanized for our convenience. One of my spiritual teachers, a feline named Bandito, was brought to me at the hospital to be euthanized. His family reported that he had started urinating all over their house and at fourteen years of age they did not want to try to heal him. Considering our sick society's situation and pet overpopulation problem, I almost did euthanize him. By some miracle that I will always be so grateful for, we decided to adopt Bandito as our hospital cat to help him. His inappropriate urination was caused by a urinary tract infection that was quickly cured. Bandito is now nineteen years old. He showers me with love every day I spend with him at the hospital, reminding me of how each life counts, asking me to care for each soul on my path the same way I cared for him: by taking the time to help and heal, with love and compassion, one soul at a time.

Some situations, like the one of Pepper, can be tricky to assess and warrant extensive communication between the veterinarian and the pet owner. Pepper was a five-year-old Australian shepherd with severe separation anxiety. Pepper loved mom but could not be alone with anyone else. Mom became very ill and needed to move across country where Pepper could not follow. After trying to adopt Pepper to family members, without success due to her severe anxiety, it was decided that sending Pepper to Heaven would be kinder to her than relinquishing her to a shelter where she would be devastated. Mom prayed for several nights to have someone sent in her life to support her and help her dear beloved companion. I became that person.

Reminding myself that we live in the real world, not the ideal world, I began analyzing Pepper's situation. I immediately saw how Pepper's mom, ill and brokenhearted, cared about her friend and wished there was a better solution, which she had tried her best to find. Separating mom and Pepper in this physical world could potentially cause the death of both beings who would suffer from extreme anxiety and depression. By helping Pepper transition peacefully in the comfort of home, both mom and Pepper found peace. I know that Pepper will continue her mission to watch over mom in spirit, giving her love and support.

12th idea to improve the care of people and animals worldwide: do it from the heart and not for the money

I think this statement speaks for itself. Every doctor must keep his primary focus on the well-being of his patient and not of his wallet. This principle is referred to as beneficence in the medical ethic code: a practitioner should act in the best interest of the patient.

I was on my way to a home euthanasia one evening and I got pulled over for speeding. The citation cost me much more than the money I made for the euthanasia, not even including my time, travel and cost of medication. That night, I learned a valuable lesson: the goal in life is not to have the most money. Money is not what makes you feel rich inside. That night, I was driving back home reflecting on how much good I had done helping this sweet feline have an incredibly peaceful passing while lying on her mom's lap. I felt so honored to have been able to give them such a magnificent moment filled with love. Giving makes you richer. The more you give, the richer you feel.

In veterinary school, I spent some time helping homeless people and their pets. It was one of the most eye-opening experiences of my life. These people showed me a bond with their pets that was stronger than anything I had seen before: these pets were heroes as they all had saved their owners' lives by giving them unconditional love, acceptance and emotional support. These pets' mission was huge. When I hear someone say that financially poor people should not have pets, I say that rich people (monetarily speaking) should give less fortunate people money in exchange for their wonderful teachings of how everyone needs love and hope, and love and hope are all that we need. I believe some of the richest people (monetarily speaking) are in fact the poorest and vice versa. Some of the people that have taught me the most about human skills were homeless at some point in their lives. They are the proof that with unconditional love and support from an animal, they can find the motivation to get work, to improve their situation and their life, because this source of love gives them a reason to live. Every pet comes into our lives for a reason, whether we have money or not. We all grow and heal together, pets and people.

I would highly suggest that every veterinary hospital starts a fund for more fortunate clients to donate money to less fortunate pet owners. The more we give from the heart, the richer we feel and the more we will receive in exchange. This being said, there are enough sick animals that need treatments that there is no reason to perform needless procedures on the ones who do not need them. I think every doctor (of humans and animals) must evaluate his daily recommendations and make sure that those are made with the well-being of the patients in focus. Don't be greedy, save resources, save money, save stress!

Here are a few procedures that should be done more often because they are extremely beneficial to the animals:

1. At time of sterilization, take advantage of the pet being under anesthesia and do as much as possible to avoid having to do it while the animal is awake, therefore saving stress. Evaluate the animal's knees for luxating patellas; evaluate the hips for dysplasia by performing the Ortolani test; get a fecal sample and perform a flotation by centrifugation method to look for commonly found intestinal parasites (we diagnose parasites regularly, even in the Arizona desert!); trim nails; insert a microchip; count adult teeth and

take dental radiographs of missing teeth that may be impacted; extract retained baby teeth; perform blood tests if necessary.

2. Well-done dentistries. In general, veterinary hospitals should perform less dentistries and pet owners should brush their pets' teeth more often. However, well-done dentistries are extremely beneficial: a well-done dentistry includes general anesthesia to allow evaluation of each tooth for pocketing, gum disease and other problems. Dental radiographs are imperative to perform adequate evaluation of the teeth as well as to provide guidance for extraction of diseased and painful teeth. A well-done dentistry removes the hardened tartar as well as the soft plaque below and above the gum line for health reasons, not for looks.

Here is my at-home toothbrushing technique: again, the goal is to remove plaque (soft deposit) before it turns into tartar (hard deposit). Brush teeth for health, not for looks. Brushing with dog or cat toothpaste and a bristled toothbrush, under the gum line, is what is necessary to maintain health. When tartar becomes present under the gum line, it can lead to infection of gums and tooth roots. The infection, then, enters the circulation and can affect the kidneys, liver and heart.

Keep the mouth of your pet closed and only lift the lip, making sure to lift it all the way towards the back of the mouth. Insert a bristled toothbrush (I often use a cat toothbrush for small dogs) and aim at brushing the upper part of the teeth and gently under the gums. The whole process takes less than two minutes. Be consistent, repeat at least once weekly, on the same day every week to build a routine so your pet knows what is coming, and remember to give him a reward (food or otherwise) as soon as you are finished! Give lots of praises as well, tell him what a good boy he is and how proud of him you are. While some dogs will benefit from having their teeth brushed two to three times a week (based on their genetic predisposition to building tartar), once a month will be sufficient for most cats. Do not brush teeth that you believe are painful, and consult with your veterinarian immediately.

Once the plaque has turned into tartar, it becomes difficult to remove it in awake patients (without general anesthesia). Fortunately, several products are appearing on the market to help soften the tartar which can then be brushed off, decreasing the need for anesthesia. Beware of using sharp dental instruments to break off tartar in awake patients, as those can damage the gums if inserted under the gum line, causing pain and stress. These awake dental procedures more often than not only provide a cosmetic dentistry at best.

13th idea to improve the care of people and animals worldwide: more home visits

I believe there is a time and a place for everything: a surgery should be done at the hospital, end-of-life care and euthanasia should be done at home as much as possible. For most patients (people and animals), stressful procedures should be performed outside of the house, therefore at the hospital, to keep intact the feeling of safety inside the home. However, for some pets and people, leaving the comfort of home is extremely traumatic. Therefore, home visits become beneficial and are much appreciated. When performing any kind of procedure at home, I would advise to pick a room where the patient does not spend much time and dedicate it to such procedures so the patient knows what to expect and can continue to feel safe in the rest of the house. Again, building a routine for procedures that are done regularly, like toothbrushing, will also help the patient know when it will happen. The patient can then feel safe the remainder of the time.

Once a year or more, each patient should be examined by their health care professional even if the patient is believed to be feeling well. It is amazing what problems we can detect just by performing a physical examination: cancer, kidney disease, dental problems and heart disease, among others. The best time to intervene and save a life is before symptoms appear. I will always remember Shy, a sweet Pit bull who came in to have his leg examined after chasing a cow. By the time he arrived at the hospital, his limp was healed. However, a thorough physical examination revealed that one of his canine teeth was completely avulsed and hanging by his gum tissue. We anesthetized Shy, repaired the laceration and removed the tooth. His family could not believe that he had such a serious injury without showing any symptoms. His family was grateful that we were able to find the problem and fix it quickly.

The annual visit also allows the patient and his family to ask questions of the medical team and discuss tailored care based on the patient's lifestyle: vaccines and preventive care such as blood analysis, fecal analysis, disease prevention and more. Medical recommendations do change regularly as some diseases become more prevalent and new diseases emerge. Ways to prevent such diseases from harming you and your pets can be discussed during this annual visit.

I believe that all veterinary hospitals should perform home euthanasias for their patients for several reasons. First of all, I can only wish every veterinarian to be blessed with as powerful and enriching experiences as mine. Secondly, your clients and patients know you already and feel comfortable with you. Additionally, most clients live in the vicinity of their veterinary hospital so as a group, we save on resources. A shorter travel distance uses less gas, with less wear and tear on vehicles, it decreases the time spent, therefore allowing the service to be financially more affordable for families.

When a pet is already hospitalized and we find that moving this patient to return home would cause more pain and stress, there are ways to make the in-hospital euthanasia procedure as peaceful as possible. I will always remember helping Fred the fish. Fred was brought to me by a young boy who wanted to give his friend a peaceful passing with dignity. We put the euthanasia solution in his water and Fred transitioned smoothly. I happened to find an empty wooden chocolate box in the lunch room that day and used it to make a coffin for Fred. I lay him inside the box and covered him with a cloth. I know this child will always remember his best friend, the love and care he received, as well as his dignified transition.

Here are a few ways to improve the in-hospital euthanasia procedure. Clients tell me regularly how deeply they appreciate being able to remain with their pets at all times. Therefore, when I help someone at the hospital, I always keep the pet with the family in the examination room. I never use an intravenous catheter as the placement can be extremely stressful, painful and even sometimes impossible. I always give a sedative like I do for in-home euthanasia, which allows the pet to relax peacefully. As he falls asleep, we may feed the pet treats or else a leftover of Chinese food found in the lunch room. The sedative takes five to ten minutes to take effect, which gives the family the perfect amount of time to say goodbye, as well as to get emotionally ready for the injection of euthanasia solution that follows. If a pet is scared or aggressive, I advise his family to give him a good dose of Benadryl before coming in. The family should be encouraged to bring their other pets to the hospital to say goodbye to their ill friend, or alternatively, the deceased pet's body should be brought back home to allow everyone to visit and obtain closure.

Having an examination room dedicated to euthanasias makes it more comfortable for the families when they return to the hospital with their other pets as they will not be using that same room. Using a special room also allows the family to spend as much time as they need with their loved one without feeling rushed. When it is time for the family to exit the hospital, using a back door prevents having to face the other pets and people in the waiting room. In some instances, I have performed the procedure in the hospital yard when the family shared their needs to be outdoors because it was their pet's favorite place. Alternatively, when someone prefers to have the procedure done inside their car for privacy and to avoid being inside the hospital, I am happy to honor their wishes.

I have realized that the dorsal carpal and tarsal veins (on top of feet) are easily accessible, even on feline patients, and have become my location of choice to inject the euthanasia solution. Several families like to keep a lock of hair from their pet, have a clay paw print made or else have their pet cremated with return of the cremains. Every grieving family should receive a sympathy card from the attending veterinarian and his medical team.

14th idea to improve the care of people and animals worldwide: make being a patient fun!

I will always remember the treasure chest at the dentist when I was a child. It was filled with all kinds of items like toys, candies, collection stickers and children's jewelry. Each patient would get to pick one at the end of the procedure. Although I still dislike the dentist office, every effort made by the team to make each visit as pleasurable as possible is greatly appreciated: relaxing music, toys, magazines, friendly and smiling staff members. Hopefully, every medical office (for animals and people) can get a treasure chest for the future.

CHAPTER 11

Intuitive Medicine

I remember my time growing up and working at my mother's health food store. My favorite section of the store was the one where beautiful crystals were displayed. I took several of them home throughout the years and enjoyed reading about the benefits of each of them. I remember holding each crystal in turn in my hands and trying to "feel" their powers. Since I was never able to differentiate their properties or feel any kind of magical power, in spite of my best efforts to concentrate, I had lost interest and grown away from them, until now. I believe that I was just not ready to receive the gift from the Universe of embarking on the crystal awakening path.

The year 2011 turned out to be very powerful on many levels. The two week-long internationally recognized Gem Show in Tucson, Arizona, has always been a huge attraction for everyone. This year, I was ready to experience it to the fullest. Having enhanced my intuitive skills with animal communication as well as with my change in diet and lifestyle, I began feeling attracted to specific crystals for specific purposes as well as for specific patients. How wonderful! My time had finally come; I could feel the different energies!

A few weeks after the passing of Shelby's dear feline friend, Sycamore, I woke up feeling I had a mission to find an amber crystal for Shelby. I knew the crystal had to be as shining yellow as possible. When I brought it over to Shelby's house, her mother reminded me of how the crystal was the same color as Sycamore's energy when I had communicated with him a few weeks before. Shelby and her mother knew that Sycamore was the one who had instructed me to find this gift for Shelby. Coincidentally enough, Shelby's birthday was just around the corner when Sycamore sent me on this mission and I had just enough time to locate the crystal. The more I read about the amber crystal, the more I understood how beneficial it was going to be for her, especially when combined with the additional power of it being Sycamore's gift to her.

Unfortunately, this year's Gem Show occurred during one of the worst storms that southern Arizona has ever known. Although I had a few friends planning to join me, the Universe intended for me to go alone. While the city became overwhelmingly crowded with tents and buildings exhibiting crystals, fossils and minerals from around the world, I needed to let the higher powers make the difficult decision of which exhibit I was supposed to be visiting. Being alone quickly became a blessing as I was able to plunge into the crystals' energies to find the ones that were right for me. My time at the show was powerful as I was guided to purchase several different stones. Their meanings revealed themselves in the following weeks as the birth of a collection of necklaces took place. I made each necklace under different energies and guidance, each offering a specific type of protection and power.

The Tree Power Necklace (to re-energize with tree energy and nature's energy) is made of an old string of wooden beads given to me by my mother a long time ago, to which I added an amber crystal. The amber crystal is actually ancient petrified resin (fossilized tree sap) with trapped plants and animals within the golden confines of the gemstone. These help connect directly to the Universal Life Force. Due to its strong connection to nature and the Earth, amber is a great stone for grounding our higher energies.

The Past Lives Power Necklace is made of an arrow-shaped fossil stone called an ammolite, which interestingly reminds me of a vortex with its spiral design. I mounted it on a recycled string of leather, which reconnects me with my past lives, mainly the one when I was a Native American woman.

The Stabilizing with the Whales while our Energy is Shifting Necklace was actually made about a decade ago when I was in college. Made of baked clay called Fimo, it represents the powers of the ocean and of his creatures. Its pendant is a water drop but I just now realized that it is also shaped like a whale when you look at it from the side. At the Gem Show, I found a powerful whale-shaped sheen obsidian that reflects the ocean's green depths.

I share the last necklace, the Cleansing Necklace, with our dog

Yogi. It is made of hemp and an egg selenite crystal, to wear when one feels his energy field depleted or polluted from interacting with other people.

My celestial friend Joyce had already gifted me with the very first necklace of the collection a few months before the gem show, an extremely powerful Chakra Necklace, for ultimate cleansing, balance and protection. To make it as powerful as possible, Joyce asked me to pick every crystal that would be included in the necklace, which was immense fun. My feline spiritual teacher Bandito later revealed during a communication that he was going to always communicate with me through the amethyst stone that I had picked to be on the chakra necklace. Bandito's energy was the same color as the amethyst stone, purple. He instructed me to hold the amethyst stone tight against my heart to communicate with him always. Animals communicating with us through crystals was a new concept to me. It only took a couple of months to receive the confirmation from a client and friend of mine, Ann, who had received the same message from a spirit friend of hers. We can indeed communicate with the spirit world through crystals.

The day after my dear canine friend Papi transitioned, I woke up with the knowledge that Papi was going to communicate with me through a crystal on my chakra necklace. When I picked up my necklace to look at the different stones, right away I knew that Papi's color was orange, and therefore, the citrine crystal was his. Reading about the properties of the citrine crystal, it truly represented Papi: joyful, ray of sunshine, full of life and love to give. It is also great to heal family discord. I stopped at this sentence and realized how Papi had truly brought the hospital team closer together during his short stay with us. Everyone loved him dearly in spite of his challenging personality, which I realized how magical this was.

Over the past year, I have also become in tune with the energy color and power color of some pets and people. While my canine friend Tata's energy is red, my own brother is going through a powerful green phase, which represents his heart chakra opening up. On my way to Pandora's home to help her transition, I felt that her power color was orange. As soon as I walked in her home, I saw orange candles burning by her side as well as the several yellow and red roses, which when combined become orange. Mom picked a fusion glass memorial that will hold some of Pandora's ashes, heart shaped to represent all the love that Pandora gave her family for so many years. As I proceeded to imprint her paw in clay, my fingers were guided for the first time in shaping the clay as a heart. Due to my worries of not being able to make a decent looking heart, I tried to object but I just could not steer my fingers away from creating a heart. When I pressed her paw into the clay, the edges of the heart split, creating an explosion of love! This was truly magnificent. A few weeks later, I returned to Pandora's home for dinner and to bring her cremains back to her family in a beautiful urn. Mom shared with me that Pandora had manifested herself in the clouds on a few occasions, through songs, as well as through other signs that spoke clearly to mom, including her scent. As I was sharing with Pandora's family some of Hayley's teachings and life stories, I mistakenly used the words, "...since Hayley has been gone." I immediately choked severely and coughed for several minutes. It was fascinating that it happened when I was not even drinking or eating. Mom and I looked at each other, knowing that Hayley was reminding me that she had sure not gone anywhere. I apologized to Hayley deeply, "Of course you are still with us sweet girl, I know that!"

After I helped Iris transition, I went to my vehicle to get a blanket to wrap her in. It was clear that she needed the purple blanket. When I returned by her side, I shared with her family that I thought Iris had a very powerful purple energy, a strong energy of an Earth Angel. Even after she passed, we could still all feel her presence. Dad shared how he always felt that Iris was more of a human than a dog. It made sense to all of us: she was an old soul, a wise one; she had walked this Earth many times before. Her energy was extremely powerful. Interestingly, one of her family members was wearing a purple skirt. I learned that Iris was a stray puppy who followed the children home from school fifteen years before and was wearing a purple collar when they found her.

I would describe Intuitive Medicine as: follow your spirit guide and the signs of guidance sent to you from the Universe. I believe it is much easier to hear and feel your intuition when you are alone. Often in the medicine world, books, diagnostic tests, colleagues or specialists will not be able to give a definitive answer to your question or fix your patient's problem completely. You must search elsewhere to make your decisions. Although others' opinions can help, you must filter them and be comfortable with what you are doing.

I would like to differentiate intuitive decisions and impulsive decisions as they can be easily confused. I find that intuition by far gives you much better guidance than impulsion. Impulsive decisions are made quickly, fueled by the initial emotions present when reacting to a situation, out of anger or fear for example. Intuitive decisions may take time. I always use all the tools at my disposal: logic and rationality based on factual information. My brain analyzes each situation to the best of its ability. My heart and gut feelings, also referred to as inner guidance, guide me into making an intuitive decision. If the answer is not given right away, I give it time. Intuitive decisions should not be forced. The answer always comes when the time is right. Best case scenario, the answers received from my brain, my heart and my gut are the same. However, when they are not, I have learned that intuitive decisions lead to much more positive results, both in my personal life and in my professional life.

I see Intuitive Medicine as adding one vital tool to the arsenal to help the healing of a soul or preserving one's health, be it my own, my patients', my patients' family, and the health of every living creature on the planet, animal or human. Hearing your inner guidance can be extremely difficult in a large and busy hospital with a large number of doctors. Although opinions of colleagues are valuable, again, one must be able to retreat and sort out the different medical options to pick the ones that will best suit himself and his patient; in other words, both must feel comfortable in the situation. It is important to know the disease, but it is just as important to know the patient and soul who has the disease because again, we want to treat both of them together.

The physical body is only the palpable expression of emotional and energetic imbalances. Through recognizing, cleansing and releasing these negative energies, we restore health of all cells in our physical body, maximizing its vibrancy and allowing it to express to its fullest potential. Intuitive Medicine guides you in reconnecting with your own divine power, with the Source, the Universal Life Force. It helps you rediscover your own power and psychic abilities. It helps you become a channel for Universal energy to travel and help you heal yourself and your world. It guides you in building a pure, powerful, trusting and fructifying relationship with the best teachers we have, Animals. We will have built the most powerful team there is to assure the most positive outcome when everyone uses Intuitive Medicine. This includes the doctor, his medical staff, the patient and his family, and all health care professionals involved, combining conventional, complementary and alternative medicine, and using any of the tools that benefit the patient the most.

As I was preparing for a complex surgical procedure, I noticed that our patient's pretty pearl necklace had been removed for safety reasons, which is our hospital protocol. I, however, did not feel comfortable because the necklace was releasing such a powerful energy. I felt destabilized to the point of feeling sick to my stomach. Recognizing the feeling, I knew I had to figure out a way to find inner peace again. I pictured the necklace around the patient's neck: no – not the answer. Should I be wearing it? Again, not the answer. When I pictured it with my technician in charge of performing the anesthesia for this patient, the knot in my stomach went away. I immediately shared with him what had been going through my mind and asked him to hang on to the necklace, assuring him that the procedure was going to go smoothly as long as we had the powerful necklace energy in our team. Facing his refusal and disbelief, we proceeded to anesthetize the patient. Within less than ten minutes, our patient had a severe drop in heart rate, which took three doses of emergency medication to stabilize, combined with lots of encouragements to our patient to stay with us. I did not have to convince my technician any further. He kept the necklace in his pocket during the whole surgery, which strengthened our team effort and united our energies for a smooth and uneventful procedure. The complex surgery was a success and our patient made a rapid and full recovery.

Here is a very powerful exercise for everyone who must separate from their pet temporarily, either at the hospital, at the boarding kennel or else simply when leaving home to run errands: tell your pet when you are going to come back by counting the sunsets. Again, pets are extremely visual. Tell your pet out loud how many days you are leaving and visualize your words by sending your pet pictures of sunrises and sunsets. If you are only leaving for a few hours, tell and show your pet that you will return before the sunset when it is still daylight. If you are leaving for several days, go over each day one by one, maybe using a calendar to help you. For example, "I am leaving on Monday morning, you will have your friend Luke visiting you, feeding you and playing with you, and then the sun will set. You will be safe at home or at the kennel, the sun will rise, another day will pass, you will be able to relax or go for a walk, enjoying the smells and sounds from the wild creatures with Luke, and again, the sun will set, will rise… and finally on the last day the sun will rise and I will be back home or picking you up. I will see you in X number of sunrises and X number of sunsets."

Shelby sure learned this exercise when she had a sleepover at her friend's house for the weekend and did not warn her feline friend Jackson, who urinated all over her bedroom while she was away. All he was asking was to be warned of what was going to happen. I strongly advise parents to use this exercise as well when they have to separate from their young children.

A few months ago, I was given a strong warning about a particular clause in my life contract. Over a period of one week, on five different occasions, I experienced a tingling sensation in both of my hands, which felt exactly like a light rain falling and lasting several seconds. At first, I really believed it was rain. My husband happened to be with me outside every time this happened and would tell me that it was not raining. When I returned inside the house and could still feel the rain on my hands, it became clear that someone was trying to tell me something. About a week later, I finally understood the meaning, which unfortunately came with a big emotional shock and a near-death experience: I was home alone with the pets as my husband was out of town for the weekend. He had instructed me many times on how to handle a gun for protection as he felt better knowing I was safe. It was nighttime and dark outside. Suddenly, something outside startled me and sent me in such a panic that I reached for the gun. Thinking that I might need to use it for the first time sent a flow of adrenaline rushing through my body.

All my life, I have never been attracted to any violent tools nor interested in hurting anyone. All my life, I have always wished that everyone could be loving, kind and respectful of one another. I should have known that the Universe was not going to let me stray from this loving path. Somehow, as I reached for the gun, it accidently fired inside the house. One would think that the loud gun fire noise would have sent the pets running in the opposite direction. However, they all came to me, staring at me and asking me if I was alright. Shaken to the bottom of my soul, I dropped the gun and knew right away that the tingling sensation felt in both hands prior to this traumatic episode was a reminder of a very important clause in my life contract: my hands are a divine instrument to do good only, to heal and give love always. I swore that night that I will never touch another weapon built unjustifiably to destroy life. The tingling sensation in my hands never came back after that night. Lesson learned.

Here is an exercise that I have created to help any living creature resolve emotional conflicts, surrender and let go of control, find peace and feel light, for maximal healing. This exercise can be read by a family member, a pet owner, or by the patient himself:

Take deep breaths and relax.

I let go of all my fears, stress and worries. I feel light and free. I let go of the need to control my life. I feel relieved that I don't have to control my life. I let my Angels show me the way.

I feel safe. I feel at peace. I have a team of Angels surrounding me and protecting me.

My mind is at peace. My soul is at peace. My body is at peace. I feel completely relaxed.

I breathe out all my worries and I feel light. I breathe out and release all negative energies, frustration, anger, sadness and resentment towards others and towards events in my life.

I trust the Universe that everything that happens to me is for the best, to help me grow and become a better being. I trust the Universe.

I feel whole and healed. I feel loved and safe. I am wrapped in a blanket of bright white light. I am a pure being of light. I am filled with love and peace.

I am at peace with everything that I have done in my life. I love myself and am proud of what I have accomplished. I forgive myself for the things I could have done better. I am on this Earth to grow. I embrace the lessons that are making me a better human being as well as a better soul. I love myself.

I am at peace with everything other people have done to me. I forgive others for hurting me. They are also only humans and here on Earth to grow and become better people. Together we are making the world a better place. I give others all my love, support and compassion.

I put my life in the hands of my Angels. I know they will do what is best for me. I ask my Angels to guide me and show me my path. I ask them to show me my place in the world. I ask to become an instrument of peace and love, for the highest good of our world and all its living creatures. I listen to my inner feelings and intuition to hear my Angels' guidance.

I am at peace. I am whole and healed. I feel hugged, comforted and loved by the warm white light that the Angels are covering me with. I want to help make this world a better place. I am a light worker. I am here to help heal our world and all its living creatures. Peace and love to the world and to everyone on my path.

I now allow my body to heal. I love myself. I love others.

Thank you to everyone caring for me, here on Earth and in Heaven xxx

CHAPTER 12

Intuitive Medicine powerful stories

1. Eli

Eli is an elderly Poodle who was rescued at a senior age. Eli came with a severe oral infection from advanced periodontal disease. After treating him with antibiotics and performing a thorough dental evaluation, teeth scaling and periodontal treatment under anesthesia, he felt better than ever. Several months later, Eli developed acute pain that led him to yelp when he would try to eat or drink. We anesthetized him to perform, once again, a thorough dental and oral evaluation, including taking dental radiographs. Everything looked good. Antibiotics did solve his problem but as soon as we discontinued his treatment the pain would return. When we discussed having Eli evaluated by the specialist, dad was reluctant to put him through another anesthetic procedure given his age and what he had gone through already. After a third relapse of his painful condition and the need for more antibiotics, we decided to try animal communication.

Eli communicated that he wanted to be allowed to bark for at least a little while when something is happening outside, such as wildlife entering the property or people walking or driving by. Eli deeply needed to feel that he was protecting his home and his daddy. It would make him feel really good and proud to have that job. It would make him feel needed and valued, which would build his confidence. The emotional cause for his chronic oral disease made sense, given the fact that Eli needed to express himself through barking. Being unable to achieve satisfaction, he had developed physical problems in the mouth area. Sharing the information with dad, he confessed to never allowing Eli to bark and stops him as soon as he starts. He agreed to compromise with Eli and to allow him to bark for a few seconds when something startles him. Additionally, dad tells him that he is a good boy for protecting his home and that his dedication is extremely valued. He thanks Eli for his good work, and then asks him to be quiet. This shift in lifestyle and energy has worked wonderfully since then, for almost a year.

2. Papa

Papa is a feral feline friend who developed diabetes shortly after his rescue. From our animal communication session, it appears that his diabetes was caused by Papa's separation from a close feline friend who also lived outside. Ever since their separation, Papa felt lonely with no reason to live, and therefore, his pancreas was disappearing, along with his mind, causing diabetes. When the diagnosis was initially made by Papa's veterinarian, euthanasia was recommended due to Papa's fearful and wild behavior, and the fact that mom would not be able to administer the insulin injections he needed. Mom called me in tears, confiding that she just could not bring herself to euthanize Papa. Following my advice, she took him home to try a few other things to help him.

Thinking outside the box is important as it can truly be a lifesaver, like it was in Papa's case. By changing his diet and hiding blood-glucose-lowering oral medication in his food, we managed to stabilize Papa. Mom became quickly attached to Papa. Slowly but surely, he allowed her to get closer and closer to him. They actually developed such a bond that mom realized that when she would be challenged by a stressful situation in her life, Papa's diabetes would worsen as he would drastically drink more water and urinate more. When mom was able to control her emotions and mood swings, Papa would stabilize. They have been growing and healing together for over three years now and mom could not be happier that she followed her inner voice and gave Papa a chance at life.

3. Titom   (meaning "little man" in French, also called "Dot")

A tribute to Titom: how a little dot can make all the difference in the world.

Titom was a four-month-old kitten with a very rough start in life. He lived outdoors with over eighty other feral cats. Found to be extremely ill, he was brought to our hospital for care. Due to his extensive list of medical problems, though all potentially curable, his owner agreed to relinquish him to us so he could focus on helping the rest of the feline colony living by his house.

Titom's list of problems was such: severe flea infestation with secondary severe anemia, a six inch long intussusception in his intestines, a very high white blood cell count, a severe infection with *Bartonella Henselae*, ringworm dermatitis, and perianal dermatitis secondary to his chronic diarrhea. Based on his records, most veterinarians would have decided to euthanize him. However, Titom was alert, hungry and wanted to live. The look he gave us was enough for our medical team to decide to give him a chance at life with surgery, understanding that he could expire at any moment.

Where there is a will, there is a way. Titom did amazingly well in surgery and allowed us to remove close to twelve inches of sick intestines. His recovery was slow, mainly because of the chronic diarrhea that was extremely difficult to control. However, he kept looking at us and asking us not to give up. "Please help me, I want to live." One hug at a time, one day at a time, he inspired us to do everything we could for him, and reminded all of us to cherish the gift of life. Three months later, Titom's diarrhea finally stopped, his skin healed and he even became a little overweight. He grew into becoming a wonderful friend, as normal as can be, and lives with the veterinary technician who fell in love with him while caring for him at the hospital. Titom taught me the important lesson to listen to each one of my patients. Again, treat the patient, not the disease.

4. Magic

Magic is a fourteen-year-old male feline in Canada who suddenly stopped eating. His veterinarian could not find the cause of his disinterest in food. When I communicated with him via his picture, it was clear that Magic suffered from an emotional shock. His ego was really hurt and he felt rejected. He kept saying to me, "I don't want things to change, I want things the way they were before." Magic had the tone of voice of a King, with lots of self-confidence, "How can they reject me? I am the center of attention." His owner immediately confessed that Magic was being boarded at grandma's house. I highly suggested that he be returned home as soon as possible. Magic desperately needed to return to his usual lifestyle before his health deteriorated further. I advised his owner to give him lots of praise and tell him that he was the King and would never be abandoned. Magic started eating again as soon as he returned home.

5. Dolly

Dolly is an eleven-year-old female feline who had begun urinating inappropriately on the kitchen carpet for over a month. Medication was prescribed without improvement. A cystocentesis was recommended to collect a urine sample to send for culture. The next day following the procedure, Dolly had quit eating, was hiding and hissing. This is when I met Dolly. She appeared healthy, however, she was terrified of being at the hospital. Suspecting that her abrupt lack of appetite was due to an emotional shock from the cystocentesis procedure, I strongly recommended animal communication before performing any more diagnostic tests.

Dolly could not have been clearer: "Leave me alone! Don't touch me! Every time someone touches me, at home or at the hospital, it hurts and it is stressful! Getting medicated is stressful." Dolly was living in fear of never knowing what was going to happen to her. Her inappropriate urination was caused by fear and stress. Her bladder was healthy. The lack of routine at home, people always coming and going, and her family not paying enough attention to Dolly had destabilized her greatly. Her body had become tense like her mind. After discussing Dolly's needs with her family, we immediately stopped all her medication, decided to keep her at home and not perform any more diagnostic tests. Her family built a routine which included lots of relaxing times spent giving Dolly love and gentle rubbings. Dolly responded quickly to this regimen, started eating again and stopped urinating inappropriately on the carpet.

One month later, a stray puppy arrived at Dolly's house that her family decided to adopt. I communicated again with Dolly to warn her of the changes that were taking place. Additionally, her family had to leave town for a couple of weeks and a pet sitter was going to come care for her. Dolly shared her utmost appreciation for having her feelings considered and for being warned of the upcoming changes. Dolly felt respected and very grateful to have a family who understood her needs.

6. Skye

Skye is a very spunky Cairn terrier with severe skin allergies. She is truly proud of protecting her mom and takes her job extremely seriously. She would not hesitate a second in barking or even biting whoever threatens her home or family. With Skye, you know where you stand as she shows her true colors. She is confident and communicates her emotions to others well.

There is no coincidence in my mind of how we are matched with our four-legged friends. The Universe makes sure that we can grow together and learn from each other. Several clients told me how they had refused at first to adopt their current pet, but how these pets kept showing up in their lives in the strangest ways. This is also our story with our current dog Yogi. We now feel so blessed to have him in our lives and wish we had recognized him right away.

The reason that Skye was sent into mom's life was to teach mom to be more like her. Skye teaches self-confidence, self-expression, to speak up and not to bottle up our emotions. The fact that mom has trouble releasing her frustration when something upsets her led to irritation and allergies in Skye's body. Skye's body indeed seemed to reflect mom's emotions perfectly, as Skye would absorb the non-expressed negative energies. For example, if mom bottles up being upset, Skye's feet will get inflamed and itchy, representing the "I can't stand this situation, it's irritating me" that mom is feeling. An ear infection flares up in Skye's body when mom hears something that she did not want to hear and that she wants to block off.

Again, it is important to lighten up the emotional load and not keep any hurt feeling inside. They must all be released to feel light and at peace again. We must show our true colors and not be afraid of expressing ourselves. Let's not sacrifice our well-being for others. If we do not stand up for ourselves, who will? We must set our limits and not let other people cross the lines of our happy bubble. Letting others invade and disrupt our peace makes us feel disrespected and taken advantage of. Skye is the best teacher mom can have to help her learn this. I really believe Skye's body will heal along with mom and that Skye's medication will eventually become no longer needed to keep her comfortable.

Let's all free ourselves from the people that are polluting our lives, with their words, their behaviors and their actions. We are worth way too much to allow them to disrupt our lives.

7. Lacy

Lacy was a sweet fifteen-year-old dog that came to see me at the hospital. That day, she was accompanied by her canine sister who had always hated the hospital but had insisted on coming this time, to dad's surprise. Dad was struggling with the decision of euthanizing Lacy. She had developed seizures which were really hard on her body and due to her advanced age, her arthritis was also causing her problems. As a veterinarian, I could only offer options of medicating her or performing euthanasia. Since both options were valid, and Lacy was looking good for her age, it was up to the owner to choose. Not living with Lacy, it was difficult for me to guide dad one way or another. Dad had a real struggle making the decision. When he asked me, for the second time, for "spiritual guidance", I finally understood that I had to tap into my soul to find the answer.

By connecting with Lacy's energies, I saw both scenarios in my head like a movie playing: Lacy leaving the hospital alive, which made me feel guilty and sad for this poor old girl as well as for her dad, as I could feel his pain and powerlessness of watching his best friend continue to decline, slowly but surely. The second movie showed her transitioning here at the hospital with me. This scenario filled me with peace. I could feel that dad would be more at peace too. Sharing my recommendation with dad, he immediately reminded me of how much Lacy's sister hated to come to the hospital, but that she had insisted on coming this time. Here was our confirmation. Lacy's sister knew that she had to come along to say goodbye to her sister. It was clear what we had to do. I thanked her sister for confirming my feelings and assisting Lacy in her transition.

8. Swayze

When I communicated with Swayze, a young feline amputee, rescued from the shelter with severe skin allergies, I felt right away that his healing energy was orange. I could see him on a fluffy bright orange cloud. I asked mom to visualize him every day wrapped in that beautiful cloud to revitalize his body. Orange is the color of transformation and of new beginnings, and therefore was perfect for Swayze. Interestingly, mom's favorite color was also orange. This was a powerful sign to me that confirmed their souls' purpose of being together, as they were both growing in the same orange energies.

Swayze's skin problems seemed to have been triggered by surrounding pollution from his family arguing constantly prior to him being brought to the shelter. He appeared extremely sensitive to loud voices and anger. He wants everyone to get along, to be patient and tolerant of one another and live in harmony. On an energy level, I instructed mom to play soothing and happy music as much as possible for him. We need to help him let go of the past and give him a fresh start where he hears only loving words. Additionally, I instructed mom to repeat often: "Swayze has a new life, new skin; happy life, healthy skin."

Although we started him on conventional therapy to bring him quick relief, our goal is to eventually be able to completely wean him off his medication. I believe that applying these energy shifting exercises will be very powerful in achieving a cure.

9. Jake

Jake was a twelve-year-old shepherd mix that was diagnosed with inflammatory bowel disease, liver disease, hypothyroidism, as well as diabetes with secondary cataracts and blindness. Jake communicated to me how fragile he felt physically. His mind was very fragile as well, as Jake was an extremely sensitive soul. He was not sure what being a dog meant. With a profound lack of self-confidence, he was afraid to "be" and did not know how to be. Interestingly, when I shared my communication with mom, she confessed taking care of Jake much more like a human than a dog, hence his confusion.

Chewing comforts him like a baby with a pacifier. He telepathically showed me a white fluffy stuffed toy that he wanted to chew to release his anxiety, which would prevent him from chewing inappropriate things around the house. Shortly after becoming blind, Jake became intolerant to being crated when his family would leave the house. The crate made his body feel restricted. Although roaming the whole house without mom or dad felt too overwhelming to him, he agreed that the laundry room was perfect as it would allow his body to move and his energy to flow, yet make him feel safe.

Everything with Jake was slow, like his walking and his eating. He was very cautious in all aspects of his life. He preferred low impact exercises and still enjoyed going for walks on a leash, although he now needed to have mom's guidance every step of the way. His body organs, like his mind, were slow and fragile, not knowing how to be either, therefore underproductive. When I asked him if he wanted cataract surgery so he could see again, Jake's answer was: "Whatever mom thinks." Therefore, I asked Jake's Angels if surgery was going to be beneficial and the answer was no. Surgery would in fact slow him down in the learning of his life lessons and soul mission. His vision being blurry went along with his identity being blurry. This is what his cataracts were here to teach: show others your true colors.

By feeling stronger mentally and finding his identity, he would conquer his fear and "be". His organs would define themselves as well and start healing. Jake really wanted to be the best dog he could be. He just did not know how. I instructed his family to tell him "good dog" as opposed to "good boy", to help him identify with being a dog, and to teach him commands like "shake" or "kiss" to boost his self-confidence as well.

Although Jake relied mainly on mom for guidance, I instructed him to watch his big Rottweiler brother, Caesar, to learn how to be a dog. Caesar was a complete ball of energy, squeezing each drop of fun out of life. He was strong, a fast eater, a fast runner, a go-getter. Jake needed to learn to bite hard in life, to have fun and to be more like his brother.

A few weeks later, Jake's appetite and energy level had continued to decline. His family was going to be leaving town and had planned on boarding Jake while away. However, mom and dad were extremely worried about this situation and asked me to communicate with Jake again. When I asked Jake if he was ready to transition into the next world, again he said, "Whatever mom thinks". It was clear that Jake was going to need help transitioning as he did not have the mental strength and abilities to break his emotional ties with mom. Confusion and anxiety were growing as he felt his body declining. He was still trying amazingly hard to be the best dog he could be and to stay strong and alive. When I asked him if he was okay being boarded while his family was going away, I immediately became filled with extreme sadness and feelings of loneliness. These feelings were so intense that I burst into tears.

I immediately gave Jake an immense hug (telepathically), told him that he was never going to be alone and therefore not to worry. When I asked his Angels if euthanasia was going to prevent Jake from fulfilling his life mission, they said no, as the lesson was in fact for his family. Jake was going to continue growing on the other side. The lesson for his family was to learn to let Jake go. Realizing that they had the power to free him, we scheduled to assist Jake in his transition as soon as possible. Being intensely important for mom that Jake did not transition during a storm, although we were in the middle of the rainy season, that afternoon was hot and sunny, a perfect day for Jake to transition.

10. Edy

Edy was an eleven-year-old feline that came to see me for vomiting and weight loss. I immediately found a mass in her abdomen. Discussing our options of performing an abdominal ultrasound and exploratory surgery at the hospital, or referring her to a specialist, sensing mom's needs to do everything she could for Edy, we decided that Edy was going to be evaluated by the specialist. As soon as the ultrasound was performed, mom called me, devastated. The specialist had told her that Edy had stomach cancer and that nothing could be done.

I could tell that mom was not ready to give up. Her inner feelings were telling her to continue researching a way to help Edy. I was perplexed to hear that the mass was in her stomach, as based on my physical examination, I believed it was much lower in the intestinal tract. I advised mom to return to the specialist to get a fine-needle aspirate done to find out the nature of the mass. A second ultrasound showed that the mass was indeed in the lower intestinal segment, however, the aspirate yielded no definitive diagnosis. Abdominal exploratory, meaning surgery, was the next step to find out if the mass could be removed, or at the very least biopsied to determine its nature. Weighing her options, Edy's family asked me to perform the surgery, understanding that I was not a specialist. However, they preferred Edy to be cared for by someone who would give her as much love and compassion as possible.

The surgery began and the mass was quickly located in the intestinal segment that is the most difficult to operate: at the ileocolic junction (where the small intestine meets the large intestine). By removing the mass, one would need to remove a part of the intestinal tract and reattach a portion of the much smaller intestine to a portion of the much larger intestine. This was a complicated procedure that I had never attempted before, and that could prove to be impossible to do successfully. Seeing my hopes for Edy diminishing quickly, I called mom to discuss my dilemma. Our options were to leave the mass and do nothing more, which would not help Edy's condition; we could wake Edy up and refer her to the specialist to perform the surgery; or lastly, I could attempt the procedure myself, but could not guarantee the results or Edy's survival. Immediately, mom said, "I trust you, do the best you can. There is a first for everything." As tears began running down my cheeks, I asked Edy and her Angels to help us perform this life-saving procedure so Edy could continue on her Earthly journey with her family. However, surrendering the outcome of the procedure to the higher powers being, I asked that what was in Edy's best interest be done, and that if her time had come to leave this Earth, may it be quick and painless. I begged Edy and every Angel to provide me with guidance and clarity.

Supported by my surgical team, I started removing the mass. As I cut through the large intestinal segment, it miraculously shrank to almost fitting the opening of the smaller intestinal segment, making it much easier to reattach. Everyone in the surgery suite could feel the intense energy but also the divine guidance. My hands were moving like they had performed the surgery a hundred times before. I had surrendered all control to the Universal forces and my heart was following every intuition received. Edy recovered wonderfully well and enjoyed over one year of bliss with her family. I will always be so grateful to Edy and her family for this enriching experience. Thank you Edy!

11. Munchie & Bandito

Munchie and Bandito are two close feline friends of mine, both well into their senior years. Munchie is currently fifteen years old and as I previously stated, she was rescued by my husband many years ago. Bandito is our nineteen-year-old hospital cat, rescued several years ago from being euthanized.

What they have in common is the aptitude to rally into health once a life lesson has been learned. Starting with Bandito, his fainting episodes secondary to severe cardiomyopathy (heart disease) had become quite frequent several months ago. They were in fact so frequent that an animated discussion took place among co-workers about his quality of life. Amazingly enough, once everyone enthusiastically expressed their opinions, ironed out their differences and finally came to an agreement about how to care for him, Bandito stopped fainting completely. He even became more active, returning to taking his daily walks around the hospital, greeting everyone.

A couple of years ago, Munchie started exhibiting some concerning head twitches, resembling mini-seizures. Each episode lasted only a few seconds and occurred every couple of days. Facing the fact that we might have to say goodbye to her, my husband and I teamed up our efforts in giving her as much love as possible. We had the "talk" with her that we would love for her to stay with us a while longer, but we left it up to her. Against all odds, her head twitches have greatly diminished since, only occurring every couple of months at the most. A year ago, when she became acutely blind, results of her examination and diagnostic tests led us to believe that brain disease was the cause. As explained before, this experience has brought our family more united than ever, and led to Munchie rallying one more time. Still blind, she has adapted extremely well, even climbing on the back of the couch and walking her way across like she used to do before.

Having to medicate her eyes once in a while for other reasons (being a gorgeous silver Himalayan, she suffers from her "flat nose" look with recurrent eye infections), we have learned to warn her of what will be done to her, explaining to her that we will hold her to put the medicine in her eye, which will make her feel better. We thank her for continuing her Earthly journey with us.

One more important impact that Munchie has had in our lives is that she sparked the creation of a brand new concept: The Litter Beach. Her senior citizen status has made us rethink ways to better help her. For as long as we have known Munchie, the first way that she expresses her stress is by urinating inappropriately in the house. As she got older, using the litter box had become even more challenging. By communicating with her, I learned that she likes a very thin layer of litter. She feels much safer when her feet do not sink into the litter. Combining her different needs, the idea of the litter beach was born: We picked a linoleum floored room in the house and spread litter on a good portion of it. This greatly helped Munchie, and was an acceptable compromise to us.

12. Angel Poseidon

Poseidon is a gorgeous and spunky African Serval wild feline, weighing seventy pounds. He was captured illegally, brought to the United States and declawed. He was finally rescued and safely relocated to live with his current owner who has been able to provide him with a wonderful home, well adapted to his needs. Poseidon's mom contacted me for help when he was battling a urinary tract infection that was believed to have affected his kidneys as well. Poseidon was urinating blood, he had stopped eating and felt very ill.

After giving him subcutaneous fluids and adjusting the dose of his antibiotic, Poseidon started improving. Mom shared with me that he also had chronic breathing difficulties with occasional asthmatic crisis that were very concerning. Although we adjusted his dose of bronchodilator, I additionally offered to mom the option of my communicating with Poseidon to try to help him further.

By communicating with Poseidon and his Angels, it was clear

that Poseidon was indeed an Earth Angel. Since then, I always refer to him as Angel Poseidon. He is a powerful teacher as well: "Respect nature, don't change it but learn from it. You are not in charge, nature is, listen to it." His breathing difficulties seemed to be coming from the pain of the world that he was bearing on his shoulders. He felt choked by it. Poseidon is also extremely empathic and feels a lot of sadness over the condition of the world and how people are destroying it. I told him that I felt the same way. I have in fact suffered as well from breathing problems when I felt pushed down by the weight of the world and its problems. I have healed by letting go of others' pain. We can not lose our energy this way; we need to keep our energy to heal and teach others, to make positive changes. I told him to feel light again, to let go of the burden that does not belong to him so that he can breathe freely and easily.

His urinary issues seemed to have started pretty drastically after an emotional shock he perceived. He felt extremely destabilized because of a possible move or a change in his actual situation. Because we all perceive things differently, it might not have been intended this way, but that is how he perceived it. He does not want his current situation to change. He loves his mom very much as she is truly the only human he fully trusts. He got scared of losing her. Others can gain his trust but it will take time. He is afraid others will hurt him. He loves children and has hopes for them. He does want to teach everyone to make a positive impact on our world.

His physical body expressed what his soul was feeling. That is, letting himself die because there is no reason to live if things are changing. I told him that he was safe and that mom was going to be there for him forever. He needs to be told often how safe he is. We want him to heal and live, we need him to teach, the world needs him. Poseidon needs to feel valued, have a sense of contributing and a purpose in life. I thanked him for saving the litter of kittens that he found abandoned in the back yard. He should feel really proud of what he did for them. He has such a strong maternal vibe. I thanked him, too, for being such a great teacher, he should really love himself, he is a great boy! I told him that I was sorry for what humans had done to him. No one should have made him feel bad about himself. We love you Angel Poseidon!

This communication with Poseidon opened mom's eyes to

how much Poseidon was feeding off of her own emotions. Mom undertook the large project of cleaning her life, mentally, emotionally and materially. By processing and releasing her accumulated negative emotions, she turned the page of her past. She had a deep conversation with Poseidon to get a fresh perspective on their relationship and a new start in life. As a team, they decided to even move into a new home, where they can both feel light, refreshed, inspired and alive. Poseidon's physical body responded positively to such changes. Mom is now aware of keeping her emotions in check, for both her and Poseidon's health.

13. Luna Tuna

Luna Tuna is an energetic young feline friend whose owner decided to have her adopted by a friend. Mom thought that Luna would be happier at her friend's house as opposed to traveling regularly between Mexico and Arizona, or else staying home alone for extended periods of time. Shortly after Luna arrived at her new home, she got bit on her tail by one of her new feline housemates. After trying everything that conventional medicine had to offer (antibiotics, three different medications against pain and anti-inflammatories, different types of Elizabethan collars to prevent self-inflicting wounds), Luna was determined to find ways to lick her tail, causing bigger and non-healing sores. After over a month of struggle to help her heal, which included giving her lots of attention, even sleeping on the floor with her, without success, it was time to return her home where she, hopefully, would be happier. Within a week back home, Luna's tail completely healed. She was back to living the life she wanted, with mom, and adapted very well to her new traveling lifestyle.

14. Brooklyn and Bronx

Brooklyn and Bronx were two gorgeous black and white kittens rescued by my co-worker Jennifer several years ago. As soon as they arrived at her home, Jennifer realized that her lip area would swell and break out every time she interacted with her kittens. The most stunning fact was that Jennifer was never allergic to any other cats. I asked her if she remembered knowing any other black and white cats in her life. Sadly, Jennifer shared growing up with a black and white feline friend who transitioned at seventeen years of age when Jennifer was a teenager. She realized that she had never gotten over her loss. Reliving this difficult time in her life stirred up deeply buried feelings. Being allergic to her kittens gave Jennifer the opportunity to process those feelings, make peace with the loss of her old friend and get proper closure. As soon as she did, her allergies to black and white cats, and to Brooklyn and Bronx, disappeared.

15. Lisa

My human friend Lisa holds one of the most beautiful medical journeys on this planet. Lisa had always been an athlete, running and competing ever since she was a child. In her early twenties she developed severe back problems. Her pain became so unbearable that even five different medications taken together could not relieve it. Additionally, they made her extremely drowsy all day long. Lisa became sedentary, depressed and overweight. The specialists she consulted with diagnosed her with spina bifida, degenerative disc disease including torn and herniated discs, and more. Surgery was not an option according to the several specialists she consulted: Lisa would have to live with her horrific condition, with her hopeless, but heroic and supportive, husband by her side.

One of Lisa's best attributes is that she does not take no for an answer. Since she felt that no one knows you as well as you know yourself, she chose to take her life into her own hands, therefore avoiding regrets and resentment. She started reading about her condition in the medical literature and even studied her own magnetic resonance images and radiographs. Her unacceptably poor quality of life was keeping her in a state of "existing" as oppose to "living", and she was determined to find a way out: she wanted to live. She communicated with surgeons overseas who were willing to operate on her to replace her diseased discs with artificial metal ones in her lumbar spine. Understanding that the procedure was not without huge risks, including death on the operating table, her research had led her to believe that this procedure could be a life-saver. After a few months of intense studying and soul searching, in spite of her own family's disapproval, it was clear to her and her husband what they had to do. Deep inside their hearts, they knew that Lisa had to attempt the surgery. Taking out a huge loan, with her husband by her side and her friends in her heart, Lisa flew overseas to face her destiny and hopefully gain the better life that she deserved.

It was a huge relief to all of us to get the e-mail from her husband that she had awakened from surgery. During the first few days that followed her operation, I recall getting tears in my eyes as I would read her husband's e-mails regarding the unbearable pain that she was in. It did cross my mind that death might have been kinder to her. But knowing how much of a fighter Lisa was, with such a zest for life, I could only send her my love and support, and keep my fingers crossed that her physical body would start improving and healing as soon as possible. Her recovery was slow but her improvement was steady. Slowly but surely, she discontinued the use of the pain medications, one by one. With every dose reduction her mind became clearer. Soon enough, she became more active and was able to go for short walks in the neighborhood. Her weight was dropping faster than we could all believe. Her mind was returning to its sharp and alert state.

More alive than ever, Lisa completed a five-kilometer walk a few months ago. This powerful journey has taught her to trust her inner feelings and intuition, in spite of what others may think; to love and care for herself as she is the most important person in her life; to listen to her body; and to believe that everything is possible. One can conquer anything. She advises to not be afraid to share your needs with your life partner and close friends, as together we can truly accomplish more, by supporting, helping and guiding each other. Keep up the great work Lisa, you are truly amazing and such an inspiration!

16. Lee Collett

When I received the e-mail that my dear friend and client, Lee, a seventy-two-year-old man, had passed away, I just could not believe it. Lee was a spunky man, young at heart, with an unmatched love for all animals. His latest act of heroism was the adoption of a blind feline named Shirley. Their deep bond and special relationship was obvious to all. I immediately called our common friend, Merry, to find out more about Lee's illness. She right away informed me that he had actually woken up from his coma and was still alive, although he was expected to die at anytime. Lee's family allowed me to visit him that night in hospice.

On my way, I was thinking about what I was going to say to him. Lee had a big impact on my life and my career, and I was wondering what kind of help he would want from me, if any. I realized that it might be too late to be able to communicate with him. I had not listened to the radio in over a month and I had an urge to turn it on. The song "Need You Now" by Lady Antebellum was playing. It spoke strongly to me and I started believing that my help may be indeed needed. Having just completed the writing of this very book, I thought it would be a beneficial tool to help Lee in this process of either living or dying. I suddenly felt strongly about needing to help him go home in order to allow him, at the very least, to transition peacefully, in the comfort of home, surrounded by his two and four-legged family members.

I became concerned about who else was going to be with Lee when I would arrive. Would I be able to be myself and share my thoughts with him? Would he feel comfortable talking to me in front of his friends and family members? As I got closer to my destination, I suddenly felt much better about the guidance I could provide Lee. At this same moment, I received strong divine approval as my GPS indicated for me to make the next left turn on "Lee" street. I smiled with relief.

Before I left work that day, my feline teacher Bandito instructed me to wear my Purple Heart necklace, which was going to be beneficial in helping Lee. I had made this necklace in Fimo the year before but did not know its meaning until now: Human Intervention. That is when I also remembered a client of mine, an intuitive life coach, Jennifer, who had told me a few years back that my work on Earth was going to expand to helping humans in a few years. Her reading and timing could not have been more perfect.

When I arrived in Lee's room, I found him sleeping with no family member present. Merry arrived just a few minutes behind me and Lee woke up at the same time. We found Lee to be sharp, alert and in good spirits, wanting to listen to rock music, which the nurse found for him. Was he truly dying?

Lee had lived with illness his whole life. He was diagnosed with liver disease at forty years of age and was told that he only had two more years to live. The prescribed methotrexate for his psoriasis when he was in his twenties was suspected to have damaged his liver. He was also diagnosed several years ago with multiple gastrointestinal varices, from his esophagus to his colon, which would cause profuse bleeding intermittently. While Lee had always known that his situation was life-threatening, he chose to live his life to its fullest potential by looking at the bright side only. He never allowed his illness to be an excuse for not going on an adventure with his family or help other people in need.

Lee experienced several ups and downs of his medical condition over the years. Every time he would manage to fight back and regain a good quality of life to share more beautiful moments with his loved ones. However, this time was different. Although he had miraculously rallied several times over the past three days spent in ICU, and woken up from his coma, there was now nothing left to do but wait to die in hospice.

When I visited with Lee, I found him swimming in confusion about his own situation. His surgery was cancelled and he did not know why. All he wanted was to go home to see his cats and die at home if this was what God wanted. Lee, Merry and I were gifted with an hour of intimate time to share different ideas about why we get sick, the Afterlife, what is the purpose of life, etc. We felt blessed, being able to have this precious one-on-one time to bring Lee comfort and reassurance that he was much loved and safe on this journey. I was trying to mentally flip through this very book to share with him the most valuable information. I told Lee that even the best doctor can not tell you exactly when you are going to die; we must be involved in our own healing and dying; we don't want to miss our exit door; the purpose of living is to grow through life challenges and become a better soul, to love and forgive ourselves and others as we all make mistakes. When our work here is done, we must then take our exit door. Is your work here done? What do you want? Do you have any fears? Any hold backs? Lee was able to share intimate fears and concerns, as well as express his own beliefs. He was comforted by our approval and words of guidance. I felt good inside. I felt like Merry and I had assisted him in regaining his own power to be the leader of his own life story.

The day following my visit with Lee, I spent time at home in my medicine wheel and strongly felt that Lee had more to accomplish on this Earth. I received a message from the Universe for him: "Choose to live. The Universe needs you here for a while longer. Choose to live!" In the week that followed, Lee rallied many times, supported by his wife of fifty-one years, Anna, as well as his daughter Christine. His will to live became strong. I even received an e-mail from his granddaughter, Shannon, who was able to fly in from Germany to see Lee, referring to him as "the well-known medical mystery/miracle". Lee regained enough strength to enjoy the Jacuzzi bathtub in hospice and walk down the hall to get his own morning coffee. What a celebration! Lee was back in charge of his own life! By that time, Lee's son, Christopher, had finally arrived from Japan. The Collett Circle was now complete. Everyone was able to spend family and alone time with Lee. Everyone was able to express to Lee how much he was loved, how much he had impacted his loved ones' lives and changed their worlds – Lee was the best poppa in the world!

Since the beginning of Lee's illness, Anna and Lee had discussed everything in preparation except for hospice. It was always assumed that Lee would die at home. It felt awful to Anna to let him die in hospice, but she did not believe that she could handle the profuse bleedings that would occur at home, which made her feel extremely overwhelmed. Nevertheless, Anna and her family decided to keep no secret from Lee and discussed the situation with him. Lee looked at Anna and told her that it was okay, he knew where he was and what it meant. However, Lee's illness allowed Anna to face her biggest fears, and in spite of Lee's intermittent bleedings, it was decided to bring him home after one week spent in hospice. Anna learned to care for her beloved husband, to handle the blood and to administer the medications. Anna learned that she was stronger than she thought as she was able to care for her husband, allowing him to be home. This brought much comfort to the whole family. Lee's three cats gave him a warm welcome home! In spite of all the visitors coming and going, Shirley was determined to spend some quality time with her dad. This blind girl memorized Lee's new bed and accommodations and figured out how to jump on the bed to come rub against him. Anna even found the strength to give Lee permission to leave her. She assured him that she, Shirley and their other feline friends, Sally and Chili Bean, would be okay.

The night that Lee was brought home, he had a very big bleed that made him feel very weak. The following day, he could no longer talk but would smile and make affirming noises to Anna as she was recounting their lives together. Everything that Lee wanted was now accomplished. Lee knew it was now time to leave and free himself. He transitioned peacefully, with dignity, in the comfort of home, surrounded by his loved ones during his fourth evening at home.

His family firmly believes that all throughout his life, Lee's "do or die" attitude was the reason that he survived as long as he did: "Do what you want, live your life to the fullest while you can, and when your time comes, die quickly and comfortably at home. Be in charge of your own life." His family is grateful for the medical recoveries that gave them yet another chance to express their love and acceptance of God's grace and generosity.

Christine had a visit from her dad the night he passed. She woke up to Lee in her room. When she opened her eyes, she saw the ceiling of her bedroom completely covered with twinkling stars that looked like Lee's smiling eyes. She knew that it was him visiting. This made her smile and brought her much comfort. Lee had promised Christine that he would come see her in her dreams. Lee always keeps his promises.

I thank Lee from the bottom of my heart for the last minute teachings before his departure. Again, I was reminded that "listening to your patient" is vital. Lee's teachings have shaped me into a better person to help more people and animals live and die, honoring one's wishes to have dignity and respect until the end of one's Earthly journey. Thank you Lee!

CHAPTER 13

Discover and unleash your power and intuition

1. Follow your intuition each step of the way. You may not know the end result but trust the Universe and your higher powers. Always remember that if it felt right in your heart to take a step, it was the right decision. Even if the step led to apparently more trouble at first, something good has, and will, come out of this! Remember that some troubles are actually blessings in disguise.

2. Seek assistance from family members as well as professionals who have your best interest at heart: doctors, therapists, trainers, life coaches, shamans, mediums, intuitives, animal communicators and energy workers. Seek guidance from total biology of living beings, hypnosis, past life regression and any other alternative medicine methods that you find beneficial.

3. Make the decision today that you will not allow anyone to take away your energy and happiness. You will not allow anyone to control you, bring you down or prevent you from becoming the person you want to become and accomplish the things you want to accomplish.

4. Share control of your life with the Universe and no one else. Listen to the signs of guidance sent into your life to reconnect with your life purpose and soul mission. Learn your lessons quickly.

5. Teach children and teenagers to be proud of expressing who they are. Ask them to share with you their needs, their passions and their dreams. They should be comfortable being. They should

be around people that motivate them to be themselves, who appreciate them for their uniqueness, who bring out the best in them!

6. Children and animals have so much potential. Help them find their uniqueness as opposed to forcing them into doing something they dislike, or else fitting in little boxes that all look the same.

7. Get to know yourself, spend time alone with yourself.

8. Do the little things well, as the little things are what matters the most: smile, give someone a compliment, offer to help someone, give something that you love to someone in need, make someone else feel good.

9. Our first duty and most important job as a human is to be a decent human being.

10. Make a living doing what you love. Your job, what you are meant to be doing (and it can be anything), may not have a name yet! What matters most is not what we do but who we are when we do it. Be your best self in everything you do.

11. Why does your current job exist? Is there a better way to do it, a way that would be kinder to your planet? Add personality and spirituality to your work so it does not feel like work. Have fun doing it! Feel good doing it!

12. Life is never about money or control of others. Your riches are calculated by who you are, not what you have. The more you give and share, the more you will receive.

13. Everything happens for a reason, for the growth of the soul.

14. Decide to be happy no matter what. Find what makes you happy. Have fun in life!

15. Anything you do must come from the heart. Whatever you do, do it for the right reason.

16. The sky is the limit. In an ideal world, I would do this: ____. Now

that you have found what you want to do, your job on the team, do it! Don't let obstacles stop you! Trust your vision. Don't give up on your dreams or on yourself. Everything is possible. If you believe something can not be done, you will be awakened by the noise of someone else doing it.

17. Live in harmony with your world, nature and its living creatures.

18. When you get ready to transition into the next world, how will you reflect on your life? How did you make others feel? Did you leave positive footprints? Work on your legacy now. Each action we take impacts our world, good or bad.

19. Remain faithful to yourself and to who you are. Stay focused, stay on your path and stay true to yourself. Remember who you are. Be the most important person in your life. Unfortunately, sometimes, in order to remain true to ourselves and our needs, others may get hurt. We must respect a loved one's decisions even though we may not always understand them.

20. Remember to laugh.

21. Take time to rest, take time to play, take time for yourself. Enjoy time with your family.

22. You are what you eat.

23. Choose to focus on the good in your life, on what you have, as opposed to focusing on the bad and on what you do not have, which only leads to more loss and sickness. Surround yourself with people that have good and uplifting energy as opposed to people who are damaging you and bringing you down. Do not give people one bit of your precious energy.

24. Love your job, love your life and never retire. Do not wait to retire to be happy. Live now! Take vacations now. Be fulfilled now.

25. Be a channel for Universal Energy to do its work, heal our world, for the higher good of the planet and its creatures.

26. Be the change you want to see in your world. Share your knowledge with others. You have the power to change your life and your world.

27. Live simply.

28. When you feel lost in life, return to your childhood dreams. This will help you find your life purpose. Also ask yourself, what do I love? What are my passions? If I could do anything I wanted in life (and you can), what would it be?

29. Remember that to be successful, it takes both attitude and aptitude.

30. Don't take things personally. Don't sweat the small stuff. Remember to take a step back and look at the big picture. Are your negative emotions worth it? Focus on what really matters in life and look at the bright side of life like children and animals do.

31. Life is like a book: a series of chapters. Recognize and allow chapters to end in your life so new and better ones can begin. We all evolve. Our work, friends and lifestyle must evolve with us. The ending of a chapter comes with a grieving period, followed by a celebration of growth, accomplishments, lessons learned and new knowledge acquired. Look back and be proud of how far you have come. Look forward to the exciting next chapter beginning.

32. Send peace and love to the world. It is the very least that one can do, and everyone can do it.

33. Do your best, ignore the rest. As long as you are doing everything you can, that is all you can do.

34. Re-set your priorities. Set a new life goal: living while causing the least destruction and harm possible.

35. Teach by example.

36. Be aware of your impact on your world at all times. May your footsteps be light, quiet and respectful as opposed to loud and crushing. Be a friend for every life you meet. In case of doubt, ask yourself: If I were this animal, I'd feel ____ and want ____. Do to others what you want others to do to you. Give respect, fairness and compassion to all living creatures. Everyone deserves to have a good life! Be the animals' voice.

37. Let others walk in your footsteps and copy what you do. This will free up your time to make more wonderful footsteps.

38. Invent other ways to help, be creative and think outside the box!

39. Make a difference today!

40. Save a life on Thanksgiving! Visit www.adoptaturkey.org.

41. Stay light mentally, emotionally and materially.

42. If you want to know why you are sick, look back on your past. If you want to know what your body will be like in the future, look at your mind now.

43. Take your life into your own hands for yourself and your pets. Start now.

44. Reclaim your own inner power.

45. Get back into the circle of life. Join the team! Let's heal our world together and build a better future!

Conclusion

I still have much to accomplish on this journey of life to continue perfecting ways to bring peace, love, harmony and health to the planet and all living creatures, and to help heal one soul at a time by choosing the most appropriate tools among a wide variety of options. Although life is never easy, and tough obstacles are sometimes needed for growth, we can at the very least all be supportive of our fellow humans and all animals, by sharing love and compassion, and by providing help as much as possible.

While Mother Earth is being destroyed faster than we can write about it, hopefully this book (made of recycled paper) can help shift the energies of the world in time, for a world still to be left and to heal. I hope this book helps anyone who works in a close relationship with people or animals, inspires medical students and veterinary students in becoming great doctors, guides the medical community and all health care professionals in bettering the care for all patients, animals and humans, as well as guides all patients in better caring for themselves. I hope this book becomes a refuge for everyone who has experienced similar divine moments and encounters with the spirit world, and gives them courage to share their enlightening experiences with the people around them. Together, we can elevate our vibrations to become better humans and build a better and happier world for all living creatures.

In a team effort, together, we can truly heal our world. It is time to rediscover our own power, and use it selflessly in a global effort to save our planet and make this world a better one for us and for the future generations (and for ourselves, in our next incarnations!). Isn't that our life purpose? Our teachers are waiting for us to be receptive to their teachings. Open up your heart to receive their celestial gifts, for greater happiness and health. Together, we can help the world rise to a new level of energy and consciousness. I hope this book can show the way to a better world!

Joanne Lefebvre, DVM

Contact information

To invite Dr. Lefebvre to be a guest speaker at your next event or conference,

To invite Dr. Lefebvre to teach your medical and veterinary students,

To enroll your hospital (veterinary or human) in receiving personalized teachings and your Hayley's Angels Methods' Hospital Certification,

Contact us:

Hayley's Angels Methods
P.O. Box 1632 Sahuarita AZ USA 85629
520-730-6897
hayleysangels@yahoo.com OR hayleysangels@hotmail.com
www.hayleysangels.com

Visit our website for more information, for the upcoming release of this book in French and Spanish, to purchase a paperback copy of this book, to purchase it as an e-book and/or Kindle, and to purchase the paintings that inspired the front and back covers of this book.

Join us in person in Tucson, AZ USA every November to celebrate, at our Annual Caring for All Animals Celebration Day!

A heartfelt "Thank you"
from families that I have helped

I am eternally grateful to you Joanne, your energy and your utmost gentle, kind spirit. Thank you for being there for me & Jessie, and for letting my emotions be all over the place. I am forever grateful to my Angels for sending me you, your beloved Hayley's precious love & energy, and your angelic presence, right at the perfect moment. Thank you again for blessing my life. "Jessie's day" was definitely precious, magical & divine.

Treva, Jessie's mom

Thank you so very much for helping us make the most of a very difficult time. Your compassion, gentleness and accommodating flexibility made saying goodbye to our best friend such a special moment. Although I hope that none of my friends will require your wonderful services soon, I have highly recommended you to all the animal lovers in my life. I can't thank you enough for giving me such a beautiful, meaningful and dignified farewell to my beloved Tucker. And I know that he would thank you, too.

Kindest regards, Sara & Kevin

Dear Joanne, we remain deeply grateful to you for easing our beloved Casey's transition. Your kindness to her and to us was a great gift. Most of all, your faith in Casey's soul...the teaching that this is not an end but a transition...comforts us still. The next day, I experienced Casey's nearness...healthy, happy, free and still reaching for me. It was glorious. I am sure there are many people in our community who have benefited from *Hayley's Angels*. A few months ago, I met a man who told me the story of how you had helped his dog transition.

Clearly, he was still very grateful to you for helping his dog, him and his wife at that time. Now, we, too, tell the story of how *Hayley's Angels* helped us. When I told our family and friends of Casey's transition, I mentioned that you had said she was probably holding on for us and so we let her go for her. Such is love. Bless you for making it possible for us to do that in the comfort of Casey's home, with gentleness and faith.

Jennifer, Estella, Sophie, Brodie & Zoe

Thank you very much for your help and great compassion and empathy you gave Monka and us. You have made a very wonderful difference in the transition of our beloved friend. Monka in Sanskrit means "Celestial gift" – that is what Monka has been to me and Secundino – and you have been a "gift" to us too. We are missing her very much and so does Lucille (her puppy) and CC la rue (our "ratchi"). The advice of letting them in and see Monka in her eternal state, I think made the transition become a positive experience for them as well, though I could sense their sadness. I felt peace and serenity surrounding Monka's passing, and for that I thank you, once again. You are a wonderful and caring doctor and professionally you are impeccable. I have mentioned you to some of my friends who are also animal lovers and have recommended your office and services. More power to you. Again, thank you very much.

Lindsley & Secundino

Thank you so much for helping us say goodbye to Wally. He was a wonderful dog and we miss him so much. Wally was always anxious going to the vet and we did not want him stressed at the end of his life, so we chose your service. What a wonderful person you are, you came quickly and a long distance, to alleviate his pain and showed such compassion for him, my husband and I. Thank you again, you are an Angel.

Marlene & John

We wanted to thank you so much for helping our dearly loved little Baxter pass on to a better place. You are so kind to offer this service. We really appreciated your caring and patience giving us plenty of time to say goodbye. After experiencing many times the dreaded trip to the office and return home without our furry loved ones, it is so comforting to be able to have this done in our own home. It really helped ease the pain.

Sincerely, Carol & Carl

Thank you for your heartfelt card, filled with such love, coming just when we needed it. We are missing Molly beyond belief but we remain ever grateful to you for helping her transition to her next world in such a peaceful and loving way. We are remembering how beautiful you were with Toby, Molly's sister, and how you were so attentive to her feelings and needs throughout everything. Your presence was almost like a miracle as you so lovingly and compassionately guided us through this painful journey with our beloved Molly. Seeing her make such a comfortable transition really eased our hearts, as she was fully embraced in a web of arms and paws, in the bed she has slept in for the past sixteen years. Now she is at peace and maybe running through the woods with Hayley. You somehow manage to turn what feels like the saddest moment on Earth into a sacred moment and in doing so, transform the energy into something both beautiful and almost holy. We are all so grateful that you are here to help us find the way...

Thanks from all of us, Aviva, Patty & Toby

Although I miss Gus so very much, I know he is running with God's Angels in the sky without pain. We thank you Joanne (Dr. Lefebvre) for being the person you are and thank God you are who you are – an Angel in disguise! Thanks,

Julie, Gus' mom

Ken and I would like to thank you for your love and support yesterday. You made a very difficult decision much more manageable. You are a gift to the planet and animals. Saw Max three times last night in my dreams, greeted and petted him. I believe all is well. Again, thank you! Love & Light,

Kenneth & Kimberly

Thank you for the card and your kind words. It was such a relief for me that Greyson could stay at home for his final time. However brief, for the grace and beauty you brought to both our lives, I will always remember you fondly. Thanks again,

Ron, Greyson's dad

My family would like to say a heartfelt thank you to you and the service you provide. You gave us so much what we wanted, and needed for our sweet Bell. I felt as though you and I connected and will always be grateful. Bell really liked you and that was so important. I will definitely be looking into the book you recommended. Thanks again from Bell, Dino, myself and our gang. Many Blessings Joanne!

Nanci, Bell's mom

Thank you for your great kindness and giving my Buddy such a peaceful passing and with such dignity. He is so missed, but we miss the way he was, not the hundred-year-old dog he was on his last day. Thank you for all you did for us. You are an Angel on Earth. I treasure his footprint. Lastly, I thank your dear assistant for patiently waiting while you gave us time to cry and love him one last time. Now I truly believe I have an Angel. One of his tags jingled two days after he transitioned. He said, "Take a rest mom", and I smiled at Heaven.

Pat & Ron

Thank you for coming and helping us with Bat Baby's passing. You made it meaningful and peaceful. It was a gift to us. Thanks for all the love and caring you show all of us, two & four-legged. We also thanked Hayley. Her legacy lives on bringing comfort and peace during difficult times. Love,

Lynn & Merry

Thank you for coming over to our house last night. This is Max's home, the only one he has ever known. I have always wondered if Max was an angel in disguise. I was a single mom for eighteen years and he watched over my children and me for fifteen years. We always had such a sense of peace and well-being. Whether he was an angel or not, I know that Max and all the pets of the world are here to keep us well and sane. He filled me with hope always. Thank you for honoring my friend last night. You spoke to him so kindly and I think he was waiting for you. He wasn't frightened at all. The more I think about it, I can see that he was ready and he appreciated that I was letting go. Knowing Max, he would have hung in there until I figured it all out. I want to share with you, again, that an Angel brought him home more than once, and last night an Angel took him Home again. I don't think it was an accident that you were referred. I didn't know the name of your service until you came. I am comforted by the name *Hayley's Angels*, and why you came to have this service. Perhaps Hayley was waiting for Max. I'd like to think so. Once again thank you, you are a blessing! Peace,

Maria, Max's mom

Just a quick note to express my gratitude for your help with Ching. Thanks for being a human Angel, and caring for our animals like they are your own. You are a rare and compassionate individual. Don't ever change. Affectionately,

Sammie, Ching's mom

I just want to thank you again for making Binky's passing so peaceful and fear-free. She was always afraid of going to the vet, and I didn't want her last moments spent in fear. I still find myself looking over to her corner, but she is not there. Still, I know she's in a better place without pain or fear. You are a wonderful person, and I'll never be able to adequately thank you. The world is a better place because of people like you. Thank you again,

Dave, Binky's dad

It's been one week today since you came to my home and helped me say goodbye to Tess. I just wanted you to know how special that moment you gave me with Tess was. Tess has been my very best friend for the last eighteen years. I'm glad she is resting in Heaven, she deserves that. I wouldn't trade our lives together for anything. Tess has blessed me more than I could ever thank her for. Thank you again. Thank you for the card and a lock of her hair. I hope you know how special you are. This may be odd to say but thank you for sharing my last moments with my Angel Tess. God Bless,

Shawn, Tess' dad

Thank you for coming back sooner from California to assist in Goldenstar's transition. I appreciate so much your words. Whenever I feel guilt, I remember what you said and the pain is eased. Thank you for your lovely card, it is very helpful for our healing. We miss her terribly. The rest of the cats did grieve for her. Her closest friend, Blanco, is grieving the most. Thank you again, and I will refer your kind and loving service to anyone in need. Love,

Rose, Goldenstar's mom

With a smile that warms and a heart that cares, one person can make all the difference in the world. In just the right way, at just the right time, you were there. You gave Buddy dignity in death, a Viking's departure. I hope the same for me. Thank you,

Terry & family

Resources

1. **Music CD: Reiki Whale Song**
   Heal with the whales, Reconnect with the Source
   By Kamal

2. Ginette Larochelle, N.D.
   Naturopath, Consultant in Total Biology of Living Beings
   Quebec, CANADA
   gilaroc@hotmail.com

3. Judy Ferrig, M.S.
   Reiki Master, Animal Communicator
   Energy work for people and animals
   Tucson, AZ USA
   520-245-4214
   http://OpenPathways-EnergyAndCommunication.com
   Various workshops available

4. Linda Johns
   Animal Communicator, Healing Practitioner
   Tucson, AZ USA
   520-825-4645
   www.journeytohealing.com
   Animal communication classes and online training available

5. Babette DeLeonard
   Shamanic practitioner
   Tucson, AZ USA
   520-256-4811
   maestro_bb@hotmail.com

6. **Academy of Intuition Medicine®**
   Mill Valley, CA USA
   415-381-1010
   www.IntuitionMedicine.org

   AND

   Energy Medicine University
   Mill Valley, CA USA
   415-331-1011
   www.EnergyMedicineUniversity.org

7. Juliana Rose Teal
   Astrologer & Intuitive
   Tucson, AZ USA
   520-404-4707
   www.HawkFlightAstrology.com

8. Jennifer Hillman
   Intuitive Life Coach/ Catalyze
   Tucson AZ USA
   jen@jenniferhillman.com
   www.jenniferhillman.com

9. Isabelle Lefebvre, M.Sc. ASCM Clinical Exercise Specialist
   Health & Wellness Coach
   Specializes in helping mothers cope with illness and live a fulfilling life
   Quebec, CANADA
   www.isabellelefebvre.com
   Skype: bebelfefive

10. Margaret Andriani
    Life Coach
    Santa Fe, NM, USA
    505-466-6210
    margaret.andriani@gmail.com

11. Mary A. Rosas
    Masters of Psychology and Registered Art Therapist
    Emotional Health & Wellness Coach
    Sahuarita, AZ USA
    520-762-9524
    www.maryrosas.com

12. TazMassage
    Massage, Reiki, Jin Shin Jyutsu
    Taza Guthrie, BA, LMT
    Tucson, AZ USA
    520-327-TAZA (8292)
    www.tazmassage.com

13. Where healing begins naturally
    Dr. Sophie Jacob, **Chiropractor**
    Tucson AZ USA
    520-891-2882
    www.wherehealingbegins.com

14. Ann Bolinger-Mcquade
    Encourages us to tune into the guidance that surrounds us
    Read her monthly column at: www.bigblendmagazine.com
    Visit www.oraclesinthesky.com to learn about personal oracles
    Taos, New Mexico
    Tucson, Arizona USA

15. Lovin' Spoonfuls
    Delicious Vegan Restaurant
    2990 N. Campbell Avenue, Suite 120
    Tucson, AZ USA
    (520) 325-SPOON (7766)
    www.lovinspoonfuls.com

16. **San Cayetano Veterinary Hospital**
    Dr. Daniel Horton, Dr. Joanne Lefebvre
    Rio Rico, AZ USA
    520-761-8686
    www.sancayetanovet.com

17. N-R-G
    Natural and dehydrated pet food
    Made with fresh ingredients from CANADA and USA
    From farms using environmentally responsible practices
    Animals live free range and are fed a natural diet that does not
    contain animal by-products
    www.homemadedogfooddiet.com

18. Dog Quixote
    Kristy Kriegsman
    Personalized boarding for dogs
    Focusing on the needs of the mind, body and spirit
    Green Valley & Sahuarita, AZ USA
    520-207-9039
    www.dogquixoteresort.com

19. A Loyal Companion
    Kate Titus, CTMT, CSMT
    **Canine massage & mobility programs to keep your dog
    moving, comfortably**
    Tucson, AZ USA
    520-977-2805
    www.aloyalcompanion.com

20. Refuge Pageau
    Wildlife Refuge
    Amos, Quebec CANADA
    819-732-8999
    www.refugepageau.ca

21. **Equine Voices Rescue & Sanctuary**
    Amado, AZ USA
    520-398-2814
    www.equinevoices.org

22. Paws Patrol
    Feline Rescue, Caring for their physical and emotional needs
    Green Valley, AZ USA
    520-207-4024
    www.greenvalleypawspatrol.org

23. **Ironwood Pig Sanctuary**
    Marana, AZ USA
    520-631-6015
    www.ironwoodpigs.org

References

1. Animals and the Afterlife: True Stories of Our Best Friends' Journey Beyond Death, by Kim Sheridan. (Hay House, Inc., 2003).

2. Animal Voices: Telepathic Communication in the Web of Life, by Dawn Baumann Brunke. (Inner Traditions, 2002).

3. Blessings From the Other Side: Wisdom and Comfort from the Afterlife for This Life, by Sylvia Brown. (The Penguin Group, 2000).

4. Earth Angels: A Pocket Guide for Incarnated Angels, Elementals, Starpeople, Walk-Ins, and Wizards, by Doreen Virtue, Ph.D. (Hay House, 2002).

5. Eating in the Light: Making the Switch to Vegetarianism on Your Spiritual Path, by Doreen Virtue, Ph.D., and Becky Prelitz, M.F.T., R.D. (Hay House, 2003).

6. Le premier des Hurons, by Max Gros-Louis. (Marquis, 1996).

7. he Celestine Prophecy: An Adventure, by James Redfield. (Warner Books, 1994).

8. The Secret, by Rhonda Byrne. (Atria Books, 2006).

9. The Scalpel and the Soul: Encounters with Surgery, the Supernatural, and the Healing Power of Hope, by Allan J. Hamilton, MD, FACS; forward by Andrew Weil, MD. (Jeremy P. Tarcher/Putman, 2008).

10. Whale Done Parenting: How to Make Parenting a Positive Experience for You and Your Kids, by Ken Blanchard, Thad Lacinak, Chuck Tompkins, and Jim Ballard. (Berrett-Koehler Publishers, Inc., 2009).

11. Whale Done: The Power of Positive Relationships, by Ken Blanchard, Thad Lacinak, Chuck Tompkins, and Jim Ballard. (The Free Press, 2002).